Taking A Punt

A Male Dilemma

Peter Endersbee

16
EasyRead Large

ISBN: 9781525270437

Copyright Page from the Original Book

Wakefield Press
16 Rose Street
Mile End
South Australia 5031
www.wakefieldpress.com.au

First published 2016

Edited by Julia Beaven, Wakefield Press
Cover designed by Liz Nicholson, designBITE
Text designed and typeset by Wakefield Press

National Library of Australia Cataloguing-in-Publication entry

Creator:	Endersbee, Peter, 1949–2016, author.
Title:	Taking a punt: a male dilemma / Peter Endersbee.
ISBN:	978 1 74305 409 3 (paperback).
Subjects:	Endersbee, Peter, 1949–2016.
	Prostate – Cancer – Patients – Australia – Biography.
	Self-esteem in men.
	Self-perception in men.
Dewey Number:	362.196994630092

CORIOLE
McLAREN VALE

TABLE OF CONTENTS

Wakefield Press

TAKING A PUNT

Peter Endersbee was born in Adelaide in 1949 and studied and played football there before moving to Melbourne in 1977 to become a semi-professional musician and teach English at Footscray Technical School. In 1989 he gained selection to the Swinburne Film School. Returning to Adelaide in the 1990s he wrote scripts for ABC radio, which he performed live on Keith Conlon's program. After moving to Sydney, Peter worked as a professional photographer but concentrated on writing after winning the Varuna Fellowship for this memoir.

In August 2015, while living in Cornwall with his partner Jo, Peter collapsed while playing tennis. He was diagnosed with an inoperable brain tumour, unrelated to his prostate cancer, and died in June 2016.

For Jo (Anna)

Family members and friends represented in this memoir were certainly in the locations and time frames depicted, but their actions, the things they say, and what I say about them are a product of my perceptions at the time, when I was going through severe depression in the wake of my diagnosis.

PE

PART ONE

1

A sister-in-law rang to inform me that one of my older brothers had been diagnosed with prostate cancer. In an annual general check-up the PSA blood test had revealed a reading outside the acceptable range. A biopsy confirmed the presence of carcinogenic cells.

'PSA test, that's something to put in your diary,' she said.

I'd only vaguely heard of the acronym. I knew the life-threatening nature of the disease, but also knew the prostate gland was crucial to men's sexuality as well as urination. But her advice fell on deaf ears, even though I had been aware of a potential problem. I'd been urinating with less than a strong stream, for years, hoping it was nothing more than par for course, a male bi-product of middle age you simply had to live with. Then, after the phone call, I irrationally recalled a newspaper article I'd cut out ten years ago, in my late forties. Medical research had found a correlation between thin build and slight potbelly, and the likelihood of getting prostate cancer.

Knowing that the tricky position of the gland influenced erectile capability and continence, I let sleeping dogs lie. Better the devil you know. As a kid growing up in the fifties, the words lung cancer were rarely voiced. It was thought bad luck to even say the C word. So it was hardly surprising I'd never heard of a family history of prostate cancer – if indeed there had been a skeleton in the family closet, given my forebears' belief in the Samurai ethic, death before dishonour. And it applies today despite our faith in the miraculous nature of modern medical science.

After hearing about my brother's plight, I avoided mention of secret men's business in the media, and the controversial PSA blood test in particular. A few years before the phone call I had plucked up the courage to mention my slow stream to the family GP. But he was far more concerned about my father dying from bowel cancer and making sure I had bi-annual colonoscopies. My father had maintained you should avoid doctors unless it was absolutely necessary. This homespun philosophy saw him through to the ripe old age of eighty-four.

Finally I decided to bite the bullet and get a referral from my GP and put the nagging doubt to rest. I chose a day when my mother-in-law needed a ride to the shops, hoping the presence of an old Londoner who'd survived the Blitz would be a good luck charm. I'd only ever had one operation in my life, a tonsillectomy as a kid. So I was quietly confident about my men's health verdict despite the weak urinary stream. I'd learnt to put up with it, as well as the nocturnal visits to the toilet.

On our way there, Sheila asked me why I needed a blood test. I spelt it out: Prostate Specific Antigen. She repeated the medical mumbo-jumbo and weighed it up, mispronouncing prostate as prostrate, a common enough slip of the tongue. An almost Freudian slip, the inclusion of the 'r' changing the meaning from the physiological to the religious. Down on your knees before something far greater than yourself due to God's devilish design in having the little almond-sized gland as the linchpin for both erections and continence – and their humiliating opposites.

After getting the PSA test out of the way I felt I'd acted as a responsible adult. Over the next few days I kept my head down in my sole trader's photography business and tried to put the impending PSA result out of mind. But occasionally I caught myself praying, or at least daydreaming in a kind of prayerful way. I'd abandoned our Methodist God after deciding not to become confirmed at the age of fourteen so that I could devote Sundays to the worship of kicking a football and riding bikes and building go-carts with my next-oldest brother, Doug. But I never entirely abandoned the idea of prayer until university, when atheist intellectuals held sway, much to my father's ostensible disgust, although he went to church more for the hymns that soothed his Scottish soul than any belief in judgement day. But I knew my prayers had gone unanswered when I got the message on my answering service from the GP's secretary, asking me to come in.

I sat in a crowded bulk-billed waiting room, trying to stay positive. Eventually I was called in. Anna's long-serving family GP happened to be Chinese and he seemed more inscrutable or preoccupied than usual, though that could've been my paranoia. There was no space for the handshake, which I usually initiated. So I sat down and stared at my knees, hoping that playing possum would work in my favour, the way reverse psychology had while waiting for high school exam results. I kept my head bowed while he made notes, presumably about the previous patient.

There was a rustle of papers, then a deathly silence, and then the life-defining words: 'The PSA result was very high. Thirty-five.'

My childish doublethink melted like ice cream under a vicious sun. I went blank and more or less deaf as he tried to soften the blow. He said we should get another test done to make sure. But I somehow knew there'd been no mistake. When I returned a few days later, this time without mind games, the result was lower: a twenty-five, but still way outside acceptable limits.

He made an appointment for me to see a specialist to have the biopsy. Which meant having swabs taken using needles under local anaesthetic. He said it was the only definitive method for knowing whether it was prostate cancer or not.

'If worse comes to worst I can highly recommend this surgeon,' he said, handing me a card. 'He's known as the "Finger Man" because he's famous for his nerve-sparing skills, and also has a brilliant track record on preventing incontinence.'

I floated out wraith-like into the blinding light, ‘nerve sparing’ going round in my brain more than the C word itself. Our family doctor had tried to avoid the sub-text but it wasn’t hard to read between the lines. The consequences of treating prostate cancer were impotence, incontinence, bowel problems, and sterility, which sounded worse than the disease. Apparently the operation itself was relatively simple in the hands of a skilled surgeon. But sparing enough nerves to guarantee even a semblance of virility I imagined as far from simple. Nerve bundles are microscopic. It would be akin to separating spider-web skein from wet tissue paper.

The world outside was a blur. Couples with babies, carefree people sitting at tables on the footpath in the sun drinking coffee, dogs at their feet. Everything normal.

***

Anna and I retreated to a friend’s holiday house in Bundeena, just south of Sydney. It was a stone’s throw from the sea and adjoined a national park at the back. There were surf beaches and sheltered coves and cliff walks. The township had an old-fashioned rustic feel and higgledy-piggledy streets. It was the weekend of my fifty-ninth birthday. I was secretly hoping for a miracle in the form of a negative biopsy result after we returned, the best possible gift.

We arrived in fading light. Out on a balcony overlooking a cove where yachts were silhouetted in the setting sun, I opened my birthday cards by candlelight. My youngest sister's card was an image of Superman flying across rooftops in the iconic red and blue outfit. She'd emblazoned 59 on the top in red texta colour, giving it an artistic, as well as homespun quality. Inside she'd written: *You'll always be my hero.* An unexpected late addition to a family of five children, she'd grown up more like an only child. She'd been ten when I left home at the age of twenty-one, the last of her siblings to move out.

I hoped her card would prove to be clairvoyant. It was certainly symbolic of the relationship we'd had in the wake of the sixties revolution, how she'd admired me as the free spirit of the family.

My hope was akin to a child's faith. Finding a way to dodge kryptonite. Cancer only happens to other people. The unfit. Whereas I'd always looked after myself; to the point of fanaticism in the wake of the hippie health food revolution, and the belief 'you are what you eat'. But over the course of the weekend we didn't exactly live up to the other famous sixties' mantra, make love not war. We remained in our private bomb shelters, even as we drank wine on the deck by candlelight, watching planes in holding patterns over Botany Bay waiting for the all clear to land.

I managed to while away an entire day learning a song. Rewinding the tape over and over to write out a chord chart and then learning it on the acoustic steel guitar. There was a view of the bush from the bedroom, which was mercifully dark in the mornings. But at night, even the mesmeric sound of the ocean couldn't knock me out. I waited for Anna's soft snoring and then her gear change into deep sleep before I was able to succumb to the miracle myself. Usually assisted by visualising 'something nice', such as a beach, like my dear old dad taught me to do whenever I couldn't sleep.

On the last day we went on a bush walk down a track graded difficult and found a deserted surf beach. While Anna read in the shade at the foot of a sand hill, I photographed an old fishing buoy that had washed up. Then I messed about with a handline off the rocks. It wasn't until the light began to fail that we headed back up the beach to the track. As Anna started up the path, I jumped into the crystalline water for a final swim. When I got out a few minutes later, the beach was bathed in shadow.

2

Anna accompanied me to the urologist for the biopsy results. I was still clinging to the possibility it might bc benign in spite of the terrible PSA readings. When he came into the waiting room he was wearing a stiff white coat that belied his humble open-faced demeanour. He was tall and dark and handsome and younger than I'd imagined. Early forties. Certainly not the battle-scarred senior partner I'd associated with his field of specialisation. He seemed far too young to be playing God to a waiting room of old and middle-aged men. We were shown chairs, and sat down.

I could hardly bear to look at him. He smiled and praised me for having taken myself off to Casualty after I'd experienced the very flu symptoms he'd mentioned as an unlikely side effect of the biopsy. He said I'd done the right thing. His introductory gambit had my hopes up. It would be downhill all the way and I'd soon be walking out scot-free.

But after referring to more papers he looked me squarely in the eye and said they'd found carcinogenic cells from the biopsy. The PSA result had been bad enough, but hearing that I had prostate cancer was like being mentally winded, a feeling of vertigo. I glanced out the window, the plane trees and clear blue sky suddenly in a different world. I only half heard that my Gleason score was a seven on a scale of one to ten. I was told the Gleason was an indicator of how aggressive the cancer might be based on an aggregate number from the biopsy samples, where anything less than seven indicated a reasonable chance of a good prognosis; anything more than seven did not. The surgeon tried to reassure me that a seven was not so bad, at least it wasn't an eight or a nine, which he had half expected, given my very high PSA. When I asked him what my chances were *without* the operation he replied, 'Five to ten years, taking into account your readings and your age.'

As the first shock waves began to subside, I became aware of Anna taking notes.

On the way home we didn't say much. Even over cups of tea at the kitchen table it hadn't sunk in.

'You're taking it remarkably well,' she said.

'What else can I do?' I was looking at the picture she'd painted on the teacup from which I was taking controlled sips, wishing I'd never answered the telephone that day. I clutched the soothing ceramic vessel.

'I will support you in whatever you choose to do,' she said. 'We're in this together.'

My apparent objectivity had surprised her. Words fill the void, truisms come easily smoking a Café Crème cigar, all smoke screens. As she spoke her words of support, I was thinking I'd brought her bad luck. I stayed focused on her Alice in Wonderland ceramic of the old lunatic asylum tower that I saw each day from my tiny office in our upstairs bedroom. I glanced up.

'I'd rather keep having sex with you as a whole man. I think I'll party on and not have the fucking operation even if it means dying sooner rather than later.'

When we'd first met, we had made passionate love in the hallway a metre from where I was sitting. It had been where she had conceived the twins we lost. It had been a strengthening exercise, if strength can be thought of in that way. Anna had studied for her second degree and I had spent soul-searching hours at this table, while reinventing myself as a photographer.

In this together? How many times had I told her I loved living in this house with her? Anna was younger than me, gorgeous, had soul and sex appeal, and she was an artist. She had taught me without even trying how to really look at art; to see the difference between a lovely loose style and a geometrically 'correct' interpretation of life. Although I had learnt to create chiaroscuro lighting in a photographic studio, until meeting Anna I had never made a habit of visiting art galleries. She had been taught to paint from an early age by her only sibling, an elder sister and brilliant teacher who'd exhibited widely and been short-listed for prestigious awards. So Anna had grown up with 'the knowledge'. Later, she enrolled in life drawing classes and produced ceramic art such as the wonderful cup holding my tea. Yet she still looked surprised when I said I loved her, loved living with her.

As we sat there at the war table, I feared the operation would be the death of the phallus, the death of the physical expression of my life force and emotional wellbeing.

After ten years I had only just begun to see why the stars had brought us together. We would sit around this table reading the weekend papers in our comfortable silences, connected by golden crumbs of domesticity, Sunday sex on the backburner. I had begun to imagine us as artists living together, but remaining independent.

***

I eventually rang my brother in Melbourne. He told me I should have a look at his robotics surgeon's website. He also gave me some practical advice that went in one ear and out the other:

Take one step at a time.

Easy enough to say even with the voice of experience. For at least a month I remained in a state of subliminal shock. Despite my family's long-distance advice to remain mentally strong, I did not feel stoic or manly.

Only my photography work gave me temporary respite. Then the void would come back – walking down the aisle of the supermarket, or standing in a queue at the bank or post office. I could smell my own panic. And imagined others would smell it too. I had no intention of looking at my brother's surgeon's website. I woke up thinking I'd had a bad dream but the waking nightmare would begin again.

But eventually I did take my brother's advice. I looked at the glowing reports about the advantages of the new robotics technology over traditional open surgery: less blood loss meant less time in hospital recovering from the operation. Robotics also implied a greater chance of nerve sparing, but there was no hard evidence.

In a state of unreality, I researched traditional open surgery, radiation, and hormone therapy. A cocktail of all three if you were really unlucky. I checked the life and death stats even though the death part of the equation was secondary to me; sexual recovery after the operation was my primary concern. My oncologist had informed us that the main advantage of surgery was allowing 'another bite at the cherry' via radiation, whereas having radiation first would preclude having the operation if the radiation failed to eradicate all the cancer, because the organ would then be too damaged to operate on. It had all started to make some sort of horrible sense.

He even encouraged us to seek other opinions and admitted that in ten years' time, robotics would probably be the norm. The overarching impression I got from other members of my family was that *life* is the most important thing. Sex hardly rated a mention or, if it did, was considered highly overrated. But I knew most men would be as freaked out as I was about the prospect of losing their manhood. Surely the magic of that scarcely understood physiological reflex was what defined manhood, what differentiated male consciousness from female consciousness. Boring old death comes to everyone sooner or later. But to lose your virility would surely be akin to a living death.

Over the course of the next three months the thought of being a nappy-wearing, non-sexual being lurked just beneath the surface of my every waking moment. The alarmist stats suggested that if I left it too late, the chances of becoming a postoperative sexual cripple dramatically increased. Other stats disputed the early diagnosis trend theory and reckoned you could just as easily go to the grave without ever knowing you had cancerous cells.

My brother's PSA results had been very low compared with mine. And although his subsequent tests indicated that the cancer had probably been nipped in the bud, he still lost the entire organ. When I'd asked him about secret men's business over the phone, he took a while to come to the point, understandable given the stigma associated with the failure of the male organ and society's taboo about male genitalia in general. We never see a penis on TV, even in art cinemas it's only once in a blue moon. Even statuettes in gardens eschew male genitalia. They're either in shadow, hidden behind a fig leaf or dispensed with entirely.

My brother offered to help out with the much higher cost of robotics surgery if I decided to have it done in Melbourne. If I decided to have it done at all. And to his credit, the young surgeon we'd seen proffered without hesitation the name of a robotics surgeon in Sydney for a second opinion.

At the time of the diagnosis I vacillated between feeling fortunate to have my brother as a reference point, and suicidal. I felt just like someone in a book I happened upon: *I felt the sick fear of anyone who has experienced a great disturbance in his or her senses.*

I weighed up my options or rather I went round and round in circles. Anna said she would support me in whatever I chose. Including Doing Nothing.

I fluttered the remnants of my sixties' flag when I phoned my brother in Melbourne to say I'd decided not to have the operation. I would take my chances and party on. His laissez faire response to my idealistic bravado surprised me.

'That's an interesting philosophy,' he said.

***

Knowing they wouldn't operate on smokers, I gave up the intermittent cigar habit and started taking myself to Balmain cafés at the end of a day's work instead of having the nicotine reward. I drank coffee in fading afternoon light, ate comfort cake and tried to read a book. But I found it difficult to concentrate.

We chewed the fat round the kitchen table: suicidal remarks, inflammatory outbursts about how I was prepared to sacrifice the relationship so that Anna wouldn't have to live with a sexual cripple for the rest of her life.

For a while we took up cards.

Our surgeon had told us that prostate cancer, unlike lung or breast cancer, was a 'relatively' slow-moving disease. Playing cards was comforting. There would be time to decide between damned if you do, damned if you don't. But most evenings I found myself at the upstairs window, hypnotised by the cicadas, contemplating the old lunatic asylum. At sunset, the sandstone tower glowed before fading to bible black.

Then, after months of soul searching, we decided to go to Melbourne and consult my brother's robotics surgeon, if not the Delphic Oracle herself.

3

After checking in at reception we buried ourselves in magazines and waited. I glanced at Anna. She was putting up a pretty convincing show of actually reading but also seemed uncharacteristically removed. When all *I* wanted to do was talk to relieve the tension. I could wax eloquent about any old thing I noticed in the traffic on the way to this or that medical clinic.

I started reading an article about a hostel on a winery in the Dandenongs, where we might recuperate after the operation. Or pretend it was all just an excuse to have that long-promised romantic holiday in one of the Garden State's rural retreats.

Then Dr Johns called my name. He had a head of distinguished silver hair and was beckoning us over with a sheaf of papers. Older than the surgeons we'd seen in Sydney but in the same starched white coat.

Over the phone I'd felt optimistic about this Melbourne senior partner who'd retrained in robotics surgery. Particularly after the Sydney-based robotics surgeon had promised to arrange a meeting for us with one of his satisfied customers. But it never happened. When we were called to a reception room at about eight o'clock at night, an old gay couple bustled past, eyes averted, and the surgeon seemed too busy to remember his promise. He also scared us with talk of 'a wide sectioning' and then tried to make light of using a needle to get an erection for the rest of your life. He'd seen a specialist do the demonstration in front of an audience of fellow surgeons and made it sound as if it were no more than an extreme form of theatre sports. Anna led the way to a French restaurant around the corner to try and cheer me up. The next day I'd been on the phone to Dr Johns in Melbourne.

'How come there seems to be such a difference between Sydney and Melbourne,' I had asked, 'when the advice is based on exactly the same statistics, exactly the same test results? *You've* never mentioned a radical sectioning.'

'We have a different philosophy down here in Melbourne,' Johns said.

A different philosophy! It was nearly enough to get me on a plane the same day.

'How do you mean?'

'We don't assume anything from the PSA. You said you had two PSA tests and the second was...?'

Over the phone I heard a rustle of paperwork, relayed from Sydney to Melbourne.

'The first one was thirty-five, but the second was lower. A twenty-five. So we'll assume you are a twenty-five. And that's not through the roof. As far as the Gleason score from your biopsy goes, that's not necessarily a definitive pointer in terms of how wide a sectioning we make either. But I suggest you come to Melbourne so we can meet face-to-face. You mightn't even like me.'

Johns now ushered us into his consultation room and indicated two chairs on the opposite side of his wide oak table. There was a mannequin's male torso that looked like a Picasso, several perspectives combined in one. Taboo nether regions stripped bare, genitalia and grey prostate and vascular organs in blues and purples, blood-red lines symbolising microscopic nerve bundles – an installation you'd expect to find in a post-modern art gallery.

There was also a large magnifying apparatus on the table and the walls were covered with the usual medical charts associated with Men's Business.

The surgeon's reputation for no bullshit had preceded him via my brother, but visually at least he cut a fatherly figure. He beamed and cracked jokes and ticked various boxes while nonchalantly holding scans up to the window, then politely suggested another room for the finger-up-the-bum routine.

I'd almost become blasé about the bedside manners. 'This may hurt a bit' and 'sorry' meant little on my personal Richter scale of psychic suffering.

I was soon getting back into my black jeans and being told what I'd already learnt months ago.

There was a thickening on one side of my prostate but no sign of a greater enlargement than expected of my age.

The more I'd heard over the past months the more hopeful it started to sound. The rest of the consultation passed like the others. Anna took notes and Johns responded to questions, even referring to my profession when he was emphasising the advantages of robotics over traditional open surgery. He picked up the magnifying apparatus and wagged it at me.

'You're a photographer so you'll appreciate that robotics surgery has the advantage of a thousand-times magnification compared with the human eye. It's a bit like this macro lens here. With all the information then projected onto a video screen. But of course the technology is only as good as the operator. And don't believe what some espouse. That only the human hand can feel what's what. I was a traditional prostate surgeon for years before this new technology, and that's a load of rubbish.'

He also dismissed what for Anna had been a major concern, dealing with any possible post-operative issues after we were back in Sydney. He assured us that this could easily be handled by intra-hospital networking and without the need for emergency flights. At the end of the consultation the specialist asked if we had any further questions.

'What about the only option we haven't discussed yet? Doing nothing,' I said, trying to blend hope and nonchalance. Johns leapt up from his chair, slammed his fist down on the table and yelled, 'I don't usually say this but in your case I'll spell it out. You've got to stop buggerising around. *If you do nothing, it will kill you!'*

After this outburst we kowtowed and I shook his hand and said thank you, feeling like a criminal thanking a judge for a well-deserved life sentence.

***

During the long walk back to our hotel in Carlton, we rested outside an old building near the Fitzroy Gardens. The Masonic foundation stone was still visible above the portico. The rest was red bricks and mortar.

We floated along paths in the gardens under wintry boughs, conversation pared down, spotting an egret pecking at an invisible worm here, the shape of a tree there. Anna's voice registered out of the void, and she pointed out a bunch of gnomes in a garden plot. But I marched away, suddenly pissed off. When I looked back she had veered off over a swathe of mown grass toward a duck pond. I left her, making a blinkered beeline to Victoria Road.

She found me sitting at a tram stop staring down the rails through the plastic shelter and suggested getting a taxi to the National Gallery, maybe achieve something positive from our research trip.

It wasn't until we were drinking wine and devouring French pastries that I was finally able to speak. 'So, what did you make of that? I feel really angry. I didn't realise I was paying a hefty fee, not to mention plane fare, to be yelled at like that. How dare he! What gives him the right to play God?'

'I was a bit taken aback too. But I liked him,' Anna said.

I drained the glass of red wine. 'Liked him? How could you like someone who plays God?'

Anna looked paler than usual, no doubt still recovering from the Kafkaesque interview. 'He was just doing his job. He may have done us a favour. Shocked us out of our indecision,' she said.

It was at that exact moment we knew our minds had been made up for us. It would be the traditional surgeon back in Sydney. Ironically, the very one our GP had originally recommended. If it meant traditional surgery instead of state-of-the-art robotics, so be it. We agreed that the Sydney man's perfect stats regarding incontinence had tipped the scales in his favour, quite apart from that more intangible thing, his humanitarian spirit.

While Anna went off to look at paintings, I stayed put. I didn't have the heart for meditating upon oil. Not even Van Gogh's. We limped toward home but finally got a taxi when we could bear it no longer. Anna went straight to bed. I went straight to the bar and drank brandy and left messages pretending to be in Melbourne for a holiday but none of my former Melbournian mates were picking up.

Anna was asleep when I came to bed, curled in a foetal position. I spooned in beside her just as described in Helen Garner's *Monkey Grip,* so Carlton all those years ago. I watched television between ridges in the bed cover just above her thigh, and surrendered to the *Letterman Show.* It was oddly comforting. His letterbox mouth and postal white teeth gave me the perverse urge to wake Anna and have sex in the sauna against the flow of events.

Without knowing it at the time, it would be the beginning of three months of the most intense sex we'd ever had. Once the decision and date had been set we decided to make hay even if the sun was behind clouds. During those last three months, until the last day of August 2008, we behaved as new lovers.

Perhaps we were thinking that if we had enough sex in the few months left, there might be enough memory of passion squirreled away to see us metaphysically through to whatever lay in wait on the other side.

But after three months of hibernation after the operation, I told Anna that I desperately needed to return to my home state, to be on my own for a while. Down in my sacred patch on the shores of the Great Southern Ocean.

4

The trip down the coast unfurled. I stared out the window as the suburbs of Adelaide blurred by. When the bus started passing through vineyards and then making its way up through hills, I sensed the presence of the ocean lying in wait for me on the other side.

I glimpsed the southern suburbs where I'd grown up, and recalled my father's last words before he died as I'd sat on the edge of my parents' bed.

Keep trying.

The bus passed a herd of cows standing at a fence in the fading light. I thought back to the big black nurse on nightshift who'd sensed something was wrong and came over and took my hand as I'd managed to hiss the words out through tears: 'What's done is done.'

It was pitch black when I got off the bus and walked in the direction of the ocean. Outside Dolphins Apartments I listened to waves breaking down on moonlit Horseshoe Bay. The sky was clear and vast. The Saucepan and Southern Cross faithfully in place like boyhood sentinels lighting the way to my refuge. The surgeon's words 'you're probably going to need help' followed me to the entrance.

I shone my torch at a security-box, punched in the combination code, discovered a set of keys, unlocked the glass door, slid it open, found a light switch and entered my refuge, unsure why I was there.

A series of framed surfing scenes lined the walls of a lounge-cum-dining room. The master bedroom had a double bed with two matching reading lamps, white wardrobe, white curtains. The cheap cane placemats from the dining table were put in a kitchen cupboard and I discovered chocolates on offer in the fridge. I sat at the teak table wolfing them down, listening to the sound of the ocean. There was no milk in the fridge. No milk of human kindness literal or metaphoric. I had toyed with the idea of having my sperm frozen but the flirtation with space-age technology faded away over the months leading to the operation.

I moved like a ghost between the cane lounge chairs and looked out through a chink in the lounge-room curtains. An apartment window opposite lit up. I said out loud to my brave new world: 'You'll do.' It was something my mother used to say whenever I told her how good she looked in her Sunday dress as I sat in her kitchen in my hand-me-down short pants before we all went off to church.

When I woke the next morning, half in a dream, my hand automatically went down to check out the pad in my undies. Since the no-nonsense Irish nurse yanked out the catheter two months ago, I'd been back in nappies. Now I'd graduated to womanhood but lucky only to have had a few nocturnal accidents thus far, usually after a dream about urinating. While Anna was at work I would neurotically scrub the sheets and my side of the mattress.

A crow's descending black notes brought me back to the first day of the rest of my life. I lay in bed staring out at a sliver of blue sky between curtains, listening to the dumping sound of waves on the beach.

***

Caravans peeked over sandhills at the southern end of the bay. Sugar Plum Island was still on guard out beyond the breakwater as I walked along the beach. I found a patch of shade at the foot of the sandhills, changed into my bathers and sat there for a while on my towel. I could just make out the coastal walk that snaked its way around the headland at the far end of the beach.

I jogged down to the water and swam out beyond the shore break, floating there on my back. I imagined Anna's face superimposed in the clouds like Yoko's on the cover of *Imagine.* The beach was deserted except for a few kids bomb-diving off the jetty at the far end of the beach. The school holidays and Christmas crowds were weeks away.

I sunbathed on my towel. The sun conjured up the endless summers of my youth. Golden days swimming, and diving, and surfing in these waters, and then driving back to the city feeling holy from sun and the saltwater, ready to hunt down the parties.

I walked up the beach knowing I only wanted to live quietly. Take stock. Spend time alone to begin to heal. Start with the morning swim. See what happens.

After a shower I made coffee and started into marking the batch of student photography assignments I hadn't had time to finish before flying out of Sydney, out of the nightmare. It was comforting to delay walking out into the old streets of my dreamtime holiday place, even though I knew I would eventually have to speak with other humans, if only local shopkeepers.

It was well past noon when I walked the coastal track, around huge boulders worn smooth from centuries of buffeting from the Great Southern Ocean and covered in orange and green lichen. A few old shacks were gamely holding on, hemmed in by the architectural juggernauts of the modern world. I sat on a bench and watched a pod of young knee-boarders ripping up the surf. Conditions were ideal. The face of the emerald green waves had been shaped by the late afternoon offshore wind.

The only thing holding me back was myself.

I looked across the rocks to the beach where the southern right whale lay buried. It had taken an army operation to dig the massive grave. The surf had not been the same since, as if Moby Dick's spirit haunted the place.

The main street was bathed in sunshine and, just as I'd hoped, it was a ghost town, the annual influx of tourists a couple of weeks away. A new glass-fronted alfresco café was on the corner where Clem's Garage had been the local landmark. I crossed the main drag to the pub where I once played piano on Friday nights as a local. Open mic night was written on the sandwich board in blue chalk. Through the windows the beer-stained tables looked the same. About all that was missing was my old upright piano.

The supermarket just down the road was now completely made over with wide, symmetrical aisles. I took Italian coffee, baked beans, sardines, tins of tomatoes, and a couple of packets of pasta to the checkout. I recognised the checkout chick from the old days despite the purple-grey dreadlocks. She was too busy talking on her mobile and scanning bar codes to look at me. She had been a friend of Zelda's, the ex-girlfriend from down here, who, even though she'd broken my heart, still occasionally rang me. Always very late at night and, fortunately, usually when Anna was asleep. But I still somehow ended up visiting her whenever I found myself back here from Sydney. She was the only woman apart from Anna and my two sisters I'd told about the operation.

After stowing the provisions in my room without a view, I set off for a quiet read in the Soldiers Memorial Gardens. The path meandered through pine trees commemorating local men who'd fallen in the World Wars. I sat on a bench and looked out over the bay. A fisherman was out on the pier. A sea eagle soared above him, and I was back at The Royal Prince Alfred hospital with Anna.

***

She held my arm every step of the way as I walked along a bleak corridor, tentatively, tethered to a trolley of intravenous cocktails. Out in the light of day I struggled to keep the grey dressing gown from flying open. We progressed around an oval-shaped courtyard at the rate of the recuperative.

'The weather has taken a turn for the worse,' Anna said. It felt good enough to the patient. I was above it all. Looking down on the body language of the man in the grey dressing gown and the woman in the red top and tight black slacks as they stop at a sculpture reminiscent of Rodin's *The Thinker,* outside the Cancer Centre. She smokes a small cigar there. Back in the ward playing Scrabble, I see her as if for the first time and fall in love all over again. After she leaves, I scrounge an envelope from the nurses' workstation and compose a poem in her honour.

Her image stays with me throughout the long night. Then her voice on the phone in the morning has me flying again. Above it all like an eagle.

***

A barrage of rock music from the upstairs apartment woke me from an uncharacteristic late-afternoon lie down and eventual nap. The white curtains were glowing. I grabbed the camera and rushed out into the magic hour. The sky was shocking pink, the water blue velvet.

The path under the conifers took me to a dark granite outcrop overlooking the bay. Reflections of light from the caravan park rippled out across the bay, and below me the old wharf in the immediate foreground metamorphosed into the shape of the crucifix. I quickly fired off a series of shots on a slow shutter speed to invoke the Angel Hair effect. As darkness suddenly descended the lens hood disengaged and bounded over rocks in plastic somersaults.

I scrambled down and found it at the edge of the walkway. The jetty was a black hulk towering above me. A wind had sprung up, ruffling the mirror-like surface of the bay. I went out onto the jetty and down the steps to the gangway, just above water level, and stared at the phosphorescence around the pylons, the ancient planks swaying like the wharfs at Circular Quay. I lay down and under the spell of the rhythm I was transported back to the pre-operation CAT scan.

***

I entered the lunar capsule and was immediately in the grip of claustrophobia. Just a Warhol Campbell's tomato soup can on a conveyor belt. Wrists and legs shackled in an S&M scenario. Cocooned in a whirring, state-of-the-art white noise. I'd told the attendant about my claustrophobia fear and was assured that someone would always be just outside the door. But when I called out, there was no response. I lay there putting my trust in the electronic eye up in control, the omniscient puppeteer manipulating laser beam levers. The voice of the attendant reverberated around inside my feverish imagination: 'It won't take long. Just a few ten-minute turns.'

Movement was impossible, the cuffing had seen to that. At least you could stand in a lift, this was out-and-out panic material. The CAT scanner shuttled me in and out and bore down within centimetres of my chest. I thought of my dad, an engineer, knowing he would never have opted for this mechanical manhandling, this modern medical hoo-ha.

I imagined myself sitting in the sun at a café where I'd read the article about the pros and cons of early diagnosis of prostate cancer. Then I started counting. Recalling the names of teammates in my Australian Rules football team. Sturt won five flags on the trot, and I'd been lucky enough to play in the last three. It took about five seconds to remember a name and number. Twelve players amounted to a minute and then I went back to the player I first thought of and began the sequence all over again. I kept my eyes shut and imagined my two footy-fanatic brothers in the wings, urging me on.

***

Storm clouds had come in off the Southern Ocean. I felt a spot of rain and climbed back up the stairs. The sudden turn in the weather had seen the fishermen off. I glanced at the spot where Zelda and I had done the deed on the seaward side of the cross over a decade ago.

It felt like yesterday.

Everything felt like yesterday. I would've given anything to have my time over, to reverse the decision and take my chances with death rather than sex. I walked back along the shore around banks of seaweed at the edge of the water. My feet were numb and my glasses fogged as I crossed the sand and followed a track past a hazard barrier and into blackness.

***

It was still overcast next morning, but the rain had stopped. The community tennis courts were hidden by a copse of twisted fir trees, shrugging off a vestige of unseasonal rain. I ducked under the sagging wire fence and walked along a path carpeted in pine needles releasing that redolent scent associated with primary school playgrounds. I had a satisfying piss at the base of a gnarled fir tree and thought about the times I'd had to stand as close as possible to a urinal without actually slipping in. Hoping other men standing alongside wouldn't notice. Now I would sit on a toilet like a woman in preference to losing my ability to have an erection, that magic male thing.

I zipped up. A party of beachgoers with plastic buckets and spades walked past my concealed position, and right on cue Port Elliot's historic Cockle Train announced its arrival with three whistle blasts. I headed off along a path around ramshackle backyards and finished up at the park opposite the railway station, people standing in clouds of steam.

There was a seat under the Morton Bay fig so I sat and daydreamed and watched the comings and goings from the old Institute Library across the street. For a few moments, for the first time in months, I felt almost at peace.

I'd been the complete opposite in Sydney. I would spiral out of control and slip into road rage to compensate for the blackness I saw ahead. Anything could set me off. But this bay had always been a time capsule. A cloud formation, an unremarkable tree, a birdcall or a rundown country fence could summons my old relatively carefree self.

I heard my father's last words again: *Keep trying.*

I'd instinctively known what he meant. It was a veiled reference to my entire life. I had sacrificed my birthright as a sportsman. I had squandered a tertiary education. Walked away from the good life. Thrown it all away because it had all come so easily and so young. When make love not war arrived in the guise of the sixties revolution, I discovered that even hippie love, as the old soul song says, don't come easy. Two decades later, during my school teaching years of respectability in the eighties, I still tended to equate happiness with sexuality. Over the years I had returned home as the prodigal son. But now, all the black sheep of the family had left was to keep trying. I certainly hadn't 'made every post a winner' the way my father had. I'd spurned his bourgeois, teetotal, monogamous life. Those final words meant I should keep trying to the bitter end. It was a sporting pride thing.

Across the park on the other side of the railway tracks was the Hotel Elliot. Known as the Top Pub to locals, it looked inviting. Zelda had warned me over the phone about renovations there but the exterior, at least, was still gorgeous sandstone.

I strolled across the park to the platform and watched the train leave the station bound for Victor Harbor. I jumped down and crossed the line just as a familiar battered grey Celica pulled in. The window went down and a familiar voice called out my name. I couldn't see who was inside, but the laconic drawl was unmistakable. I looked in through the passenger window. It was my former young musical partner from a decade and a half ago. He looked the same, draped over the wheel as relaxed as a cat.

He grinned his endearingly wrinkled grin and got out and walked around. We hugged Italian-style. I'd known his oldest brother at Flinders University and then in the Carlton rock-music scene. Which was where, years later, I also got to know this wunderkind, the youngest of a musically talented family. He coincidentally left Melbourne at the same as I had in the early nineties, and for the same reason. We had both come home because our fathers were on the way out. He lived in a caravan at his mum's place and joined my piano gig at the other pub for the best part of a year. His guitar playing and singing were the perfect foil for my country stuff. Women metaphorically died in their tracks upon hearing him and seeing his soulful brown eyes, Native American cheekbones, and scrawny, ramshackle nobility. He'd been drinking quite heavily when I knew him, mostly just cans of beer, but I'd heard on the grapevine he'd been ill over the last few years. It was as if he had chosen a slow form of suicide. When I'd known him he used to wander around the district like a young Zen sage. Often turned up at the potter's place where I first lived before I moved in with Zelda. It was her old car he was now driving. We used to party on at her place, and I'd also run into him at various kitchen tables around the district where he'd be entertaining without even trying. You always felt better from having been in his kind presence, although he managed to make it seem the other way round.

We stood in the road behind the Celica, unexpectedly in each other's company again. He was one of the few I didn't mind running into during my solitude, my attempt at staying incognito. He looked better than I'd ever seen him, almost glowing, as he told me how he'd turned his life around. He had given up drinking, apart from the odd shandy, and was working at a community centre as musical director of a band of ex-alcoholics, former drug abusers, and unemployed locals. He was about to pick up the minibus to take his charges around the district to see the Christmas decorations before heading to the Life Saving Club for the sausage sizzle. He invited me around to his new digs to hear the recordings he'd produced with the community band. So I hopped in.

He was living in a shed lined with insulation in someone's backyard while they were away for a year. It was full of equipment and instruments. He played me tracks from the album he'd produced with the band. He was perfect for the job. He had a rapport with these people. They trusted him. He said he had to be careful not to step over the line.

He lit up a tailor-made cigarette. 'I love the job, Endo. I've never been so happy in my life. I've got a girlfriend.'

He told me about this new girl who sounded like the real deal. He was now swimming laps in a pool, and planned to do a TAFE course so he could be officially employed.

I left him listening to a short CD I'd recorded with my music partner in Sydney, and went out onto the balcony and stood in the sun, debating whether to ask him for a fag and tell him about the operation, the real reason I was back down here. It remained on the tip of my tongue for a few minutes, but then

I thought better of it. I asked if he was going to the open mic night. When he said he might, I got the impression he wouldn't be there. He dropped me back at the shops before driving on to pick up the minibus.

I walked along the back streets past heritage sandstone buildings and found myself back at the Top Pub, staring in through the tinted glass. My reflection through the glass darkly brought to mind the man who came here on summer holidays after teaching in Melbourne. When surfing in the Southern Ocean and a counter tea of fish and chips followed by a cold beer, with the sniff of a holiday love affair in the offing, defined happiness, if not the meaning of life itself. I pulled myself away from reflections, and walked to the post office a few doors down to send off the student assignments in the backpack.

The building was turn-of-the-century with an archetypal country-post-office feel. Worn bluestone steps, high windows, golden woodwork, green linoleum counter and a postmaster who'd merged with his parcels and stationery, still on the job after all these years. His face lit up in a smile.

'Merry Christmas, old son, where are we now and what are we doing?' I should have smelt a rat at the use of the royal we.

'Hi, mate, and a merry Christmas to you too. I've been in Sydney for the past ten years. I'm a commercial photographer now of all things.'

'A photographer! You're a hard man to keep up with. We used to go and watch you play when we lived around the corner from the Unley Oval in the sixties.'

The flashback leapfrogged forty years in one fell swoop. It was as if my time here as a musician hadn't registered at all. It was the image of the nineteen-year-old footballer that was indelibly etched.

I grinned, and plonked the assignments on the counter: 'Will it take Express Post to get this to Sydney by the end of the week?'

'Those were the days, hey?' he said, dumping the package on his weighing machine.

The interior of the Hotel Elliot had been made over, just as Zelda warned. It was now open plan. Wide-screen televisions and a TAB had replaced the posters and party snapshots. I went out to an empty beer garden, chose the only wooden table among new chic chrome constructions with tiny circular tops, and toasted a merry Christmas and happy New Year to my now not so young former soul mate. I took a delicious sip of late-afternoon white wine. It was comforting letting thoughts move as slowly as the pink and white clouds across the western sky, drifting back to a musician in Carlton who'd been my muse in the eighties after I contracted genital herpes. When I thought *that* was the end of the world. I remembered her saying straight up, 'It's the worst. It always breaks out when you least need it.' Then she'd softened the blunt honesty by telling me that in a year or so it would get less frequent and eventually remain dormant. She'd had it for years, not to mention a long history of serious illness, including hepatitis and a collapsed lung. She was a junky when smack was akin to a fashion statement, the red badge of courage for rock stars. I imagined what my friend would've said if I mentioned penile injections to her. She rubbed shoulders with the outsiders of society, with the nightlife. I imagined her tough, laconic approach. She'd probably say, 'There could be worse things to look forward to.' It was the same attitude she had whenever she faced another health setback.

'They're bound to find a new drug sometime,' she'd once said to me, with her toothy grin. She worked at the rate of someone who believed every day to be her last.

5

The Dolphins felt more like a prison than a refuge when I returned to a mess of books and papers and wilted wild lavender in the glass on the table. I put on the kettle and stared out the kitchen louvres. No birdsong from the pines at the back, but at least I had my freedom from the prying eyes of the world. The world of doctors and family and friends who wanted me to believe that everything would be as it once was.

***

I floated back to Sydney, back to Anna. Imagined her at the kitchen table. The table at which we'd conducted many postmortems over the course of the past year. It would have taken its toll. She was a woman with a capacity for compassion for society's outsiders, always forking out for The Big Issue while I tended to walk by. She believed in community action and was one of the first to attend the rallies and meetings to protest against developers wanting to destroy Callan Park Mental Hospital and associated community environs. I had helped out as a photographer on those local campaigns but avoided the mass demos after my experience of marching in the sixties.

Her students at TAFE loved her, which had nothing to do with politics or academic qualifications. She was one of those rare people with the ability to help those lacking confidence find their voice. I felt like ringing her but we had an unspoken agreement. She needed a complete break too. The past six months had been really heavy, as Neil from *The Young Ones* used to say.

I glanced at the book she'd given me for Christmas, *Journal of a Solitude,* the memoir of a venerable feminist and poet who'd become a solitary. I imagined Anna zoning out on a crossword puzzle or engrossed in a novel. Whenever we had guests she would cover the kitchen table with an Indian sari. But the only visitor we'd had this year, as if I'd hexed the place, was a former colleague of mine from English teaching days.

Julian's surprise return from overseas had seemed like a good excuse to party on and pretend nothing had changed. On his way over in a taxi he'd rung to see what he should bring. I suggested a bottle of red and some cigars. I must've still been hoping for a miracle. Everything would return to normal, mind over matter. When he arrived, we went onto the balcony by the kitchen that looked out over the backyard. The giant avocado tree overhanging the balcony sheltered us, out in the night. He regaled us with his tales of women problems as we drank and smoked. The soiree was interrupted when the tortoiseshell cat appeared on the stairs with a mouse's tail sticking out between her teeth. We all jumped up as Puss headed back down into the jungle. I snapped on the balcony light, and we flailed around in the weeds looking for the bad cat.

We eventually found her and tried coaxing her into dropping the prey. Julian suggested water. So I picked her up and held her by the scruff of the neck as he doused her from a saucepan. She dropped her gift at our feet. Amazingly, the mouse scurried back into the garden.

The party continued. Out of the blue Anna announced that a work colleague had given her a number I might be interested in calling, an expert on prostate cancer. Though the cigars burnt just as brightly the conversation turned serious. Julian told us about a benign enlargement that slowed his urinating. But it wasn't going to kill him, or threaten his manhood. He agreed with my partying-on philosophy, no doubt trying to make light of my PSA result to try and keep my spirits up. He told us about the fluid-balancing properties of a mixture of water and fruit juice he had with him in a plastic bottle, which he claimed was good for hydration. But he also sipped away at a stubby of beer to keep up appearances. I decided to get it over with and went inside to ring the so-called expert in private.

The voice on the other end of the line was apologetic. He said he was the president of what sounded like a secret society, he'd understand if I didn't want to talk about it. He'd had the operation in the bad old days. He told me it was a serious disease. He'd been impotent ever since the operation. But after he'd had a prosthesis inserted in his scrotum, his sex life had never been better – apart from his wife being the initiator these days. He also told me not to cross my bridges. At that stage I didn't know the result of the biopsy. Despite his good intent I made the mistake of giving him the reins and he never let go. He succeeded in scaring the living daylights out of me. I eventually managed to hang up and went back outside to rejoin what had become a party for two. I didn't say much when Anna asked how it went. But after she'd gone to bed, I began to talk about it with Julian. He mentioned a Hemingway novel about bullfighting, in which the protagonist is impotent due to a war injury but in love with his nurse. I had vague recollections of *The Sun Also Rises* from university, but more about the bullfighting than the ultimate fate of the impotent anti-hero. A week later I spoke to Julian on a bad international line. He recalled the ashen look on my face that night. He said when I rejoined the party he'd known the party was over.

***

I drew the curtains in the bedroom, folded back the white doona and undressed, leaving on the white jocks I'd bought myself as a Christmas present. After wearing black to hide incriminating urine stains the new white pair were to highlight any developments down there. I was the same about women's underwear. Instead of traditional black associated with sex and death, I'd always preferred pudenda in translucent white, with the erotic hint of pubic hair.

I wheeled the television in from the lounge room and plugged in as a foil from trying too hard. The mere thought of mid-afternoon masturbation would once have been enough to start arousal. I touched my penis and, to kick-start the thing, concentrated on the mound of Venus in archetypal silken white panties. But there was nothing. I flicked at my useless flesh until there was a swelling. I whipped it against tightened stomach muscles, aware of the pelvic-floor muscles as a sort of new erogenous zone from the daily exercise to avoid incontinence. I knelt over a pillow, and finally came. The surgeon had told me it was possible to have an orgasm without an erection but it would be dry. What he hadn't mentioned was the new post-orgasmic ache, which fortunately couldn't stop me heading towards sleep. I thought about my Irish mother's approach to life: *You'll do.*

I woke still in a dream. Anna's pubes shaved bald. She had been attempting fellatio on my flaccid dick. Then my face was buried in her bald mound like a baby at the breast. I panicked. I had no idea where I was. No memory, just a nightmarish claustrophobic feeling of not knowing where I was. I got up and groped for something familiar. After stumbling into the curtains I found the door and a light switch. It was just after eight o'clock. I'd slept for hours. I thought about the open mic night. Testing my toes in a brave new world and maybe running into Zelda.

***

Through the windows the bar looked crowded for a mid-week night. I hesitated in the foyer. It was a risk returning to the site of my former rural glory days, and hardly the stuff of a pilgrimage into solitude. But I went in with the blinkers firmly in place, straight up to the bar.

I bought a glass of wine and took it over to a table where the piano once stood. I watched a combo setting up down the other end of the room, drinking the wine too quickly, aware of the collective hum of local camaraderie that seemed unique to country pubs.

I was finally off the doctors' radar, the intrusive hands, check-ups, test results, and never-ending appointments. No longer a prisoner on parole with an electronic wristband. Here in my old stamping grounds, I could observe from the other side of the fishbowl. Simply vanish off their map. But I was also conscious of a schism. On the one hand I was the fly on the wall instead of the musician who'd once performed in this very bar, and on the other I was the protagonist in the horror movie called *The Fly.* Trapped inside an insect's body with a tiny human head screaming out for help, a tiny voice inaudible to normal humans.

But at least I was away from sonorous Sydney's glitterati and rat-race of traffic, and claustrophobic tunnels. Down here on the shore of the Great Southern Ocean I felt a long way away from those cancer clinics. It was philosophically possible it had never happened because not another soul in this place knew. I felt strangely alive in my faded dinner jacket, thick black Woody Allen glasses, and the disguise of the attrition of the fifteen years since last I was here.

***

I thought about the nightmare, waking up from the anaesthesia when I'd celebrated being back in the land of the living, and watching Australian Rules football on television in the public ward. Carrying on triumphant conversations with concerned interstate family members, juggling the bedside phone and the mobile phone. When the anaesthetic wore off, Sister Morphine was on tap, turning nightmare into dream. Then, when the television suddenly went blank and the tears came, surrounded by snoring and the squeak of nurses' shoes along corridors, it finally dawned that I'd allowed it to happen. There was an evil presence in the room that night; what was done was done. But then the black nurse had comforted me, and in the morning a nurse told me that her husband had also been operated on by my surgeon. Only a couple of months out from the op and he was no longer incontinent, and already back on the golf course. She said the word was out in the medical world about this young doctor's statistics. He had set up a clinic in the western suburbs, in Bankstown, to cater for poorer people. I already knew about that, because Bankstown was where I'd had the biopsy. I was tremendously buoyed by her thoughtful words first thing in the morning. To hear her sing my surgeon's praises and give me her professional if personally biased opinion. The black nurse on night duty must've been the bush telegraph about my shedding of tears in the night. Or she may have been an archetypal dream figure. I thought I glimpsed her in Balmain a few days later, my catheter still firmly in place. I was resting against a pole just after a concerned member of the pubic, who'd said she was an ex-nurse, asked if I was okay. When I made eye contact with my black angel, she vanished into the pedestrian crowd.

Jillie Roper was over by the bar. She had shades of Joni Mitchell about her. She could have put bums on seats if given half a chance. Then out of the blue, the local with the angelic voice had become a lesbian. She was leaning against a pillar in intimate conversation with her female companion. The once-long blonde hair was now grey, and as short as a boy's. They were surrounded by a group of people fanning out from the bar. I left my dinner jacket to mark my territory and went over.

She smiled and held out her arms like the Pope about to grant absolution for sins of the past. We hugged and kissed on the lips.

'I thought I recognised the guy sitting all alone over there. Haven't seen you in ages.'

She introduced me to her partner, a handsome younger woman with blonde hair. We shook hands and I offered to get drinks all round. As I started making my way through the crowd, a couple of callow youths blocked my way, smirking. I had the feeling they'd seen me with the lesbians. This was still Hicksville in some respects. But their supercilious masks melted as I kept going, making a beeline for the bar, straight through them. I felt more the sexual outsider, if that's possible. As I took the drinks back, there was no further suggestion of aggro.

'Are you going to have a play tonight?' Jillie said. 'You can borrow my guitar if you want.'

She invited me to have a joint with her outside the pub. I hadn't smoked dope in years because it tended to make me paranoid in public. But I followed her out through the beer garden. Locals were hunkered down at the same old tables, smoking away. Gum trees and barns and rooftops were outlined against a country-clear night sky. We went to the car park and got into her old station wagon. Jillie produced a small joint and lit up and passed it to me. A couple of drags later and I was paranoid about my meaningless future. She sensed the impasse and put Van Morrison on, fortunately not 'Moon Dance', which would have been an instant downer. It was anything but a 'fantabulous night to make romance'. But it felt okay listening to 'It Stoned Me': county fairs and fishing rods, hitching and getting yourself in mountain streams, I was happy enough to let the water run all over me.

She asked if I was still playing and I told her I'd done a couple of gigs in Sydney with an old friend. After more small talk, I decided to spill the beans.

'Actually, it's been a pretty rough year. And music is probably the main contributing cause – as much as being a temporary saviour. Depending how far back you go.'

'Sorry, you've lost me,' she said.

I was thinking that all the drinking and debauchery in the rock 'n' roll scene had contributed to my problem. As well as the partying down here when I should've been looking after my middle-aged health, getting annual check-ups as my sensible brother had done.

I wasn't sure why I was suddenly confessing to a woman I hadn't seen for thirteen years.

'What I'm about to say is strictly confidential, Jillie.'

'You've got me really worried now,' she said.

'You've probably already guessed.'

She had a last toke on the roach. 'There's only one thing I can think of. But I'd rather not guess. Spit it out, china plate.'

A young couple walked past, locked in a passionate embrace, headed for the back of a car by the look of it.

'I was diagnosed with PC in March. Not political correctness, prostate cancer. I decided to get checked out after I heard an older brother of mine had been diagnosed with it. I had the operation in August.'

'Ahh,' Jillie said. 'Have you got a girlfriend up in Sydney?'

'Anna. We've been together for ten years but I'm worried about the future, if worse comes to worst.'

She didn't say anything.

'I think my recent music comeback has been a way of denying what's happened. I played with a catheter up my dick and a urine bag strapped to my thigh, wrangling tubes and nozzles in filthy hotel toilets.'

'I'd count my blessings you've got Anna,' she said. 'Are you OK now?'

In one of my first appointments with my surgeon after the diagnosis, I was told the statistical window of opportunity for erections returning after the operation is two years. I had the terrifying thought my erections might *never* return, and all the medical help in the world would not put Humpty back together again. But at least the two-year window of opportunity gave me something to cling to.

'Ask me again in about eighteen months, when Mother

Nature apparently shuts down for good.'

She kissed me on the cheek.

'Your secret's safe with me. We should go in. My name will be coming up.'

I rescued my dinner jacket and moved to another table to watch the south coast angel perform. Zelda was nowhere to be seen, probably a good thing. Nothing would ever match those Friday nights in the front bar, when the local musicians would roll up around midnight after we'd finished our gig. When the piano would be pushed into the back dining area and we would jam long after legal closing time. Back then I had total self-belief in singing country blues songs, personalising the mistakes I'd made in my own life, to tunes such as 'Tonight The Bottle Let Me Down'.

A cornucopia of flowers on the piano greeted me one night after I'd driven down from Adelaide. I hadn't even realised it was the anniversary of the gig. The publican himself had been responsible for the flowers. The bar girls got up on the bar and threw coasters into the crowd, whooping it up mock country-hick style. When my young partner sang 'I Still Haven't Found What I'm Looking For' they all histrionically pointed at their chests. His high register took the whole gig up a notch or two. I sat hunched over the ivories, having a breather from singing. Then Zelda arrived, late as usual, to scare off any would-be competition.

I listened to Jillie, and found myself craving the exhilaration I felt after performing, and going back to Zelda's, to the old house by the sea, where we partied on until dawn and made love and woke up late on Saturday, and I'd head to Knights Beach to bodysurf the cobwebs away.

It was drizzling by the time I headed down The Strand to the music of waves breaking on the beach. I decided to brace myself with a nightcap at the Top Pub before going around to Zelda's. I went in through the secret Locals Only entrance, and ended up in the old part of the front bar. It looked the same as years ago except for a dark-wooden plaque on the wall. The homespun notice read: 'Ian's Corner'. I wished I'd known. I would've come to his funeral. I'd often had the pleasure of being bailed up here by the former ABC announcer during the Zelda era. Even in his retirement years, Ian had stood out from the crowd, always occupying the same spot at the bar, entertaining the barflies with his eloquence and theatrical charm.

I took the stool directly under the plaque and ordered a brandy in his honour, remembering how he hated the lack of the poetic spirit in the modern world exemplified by the commercialisation of spellings such as 'BI-LO'. And how being still new to the area he would fill me in if I forgot the name of the supermarket.

'Oh! You mean BI-LO? It's *obscene!*' he loved to say, projecting disdain with the gorgeous tones of his former ABC radio announcer's voice mixed with a hint of camp double entendre.

Zelda's back gate was still hanging off its hinges. There was a light at the kitchen window. She was a night owl. I went down the side of the house. A flash of silver water greeted me as the moon sailed forth between clouds. I needed late night company and Zelda more than fitted the bill. The rambling back lawn was familiar underfoot. I'd once been naïve enough to believe this place could be my final home, after years of being a butterfly, as my father described me on more than one occasion.

The barren apple tree was still standing but the kidney-shaped coffee table beneath it was missing. It had been the altar around which we smoked and drank and communed with the night spirits. I could still see the flash of her thigh in the moonlight as she squatted on the lawn to take a piss.

I perched on the only unbroken slat of the garden seat, and flashed onto the night I'd sat out here recovering after walking in on Zelda receiving a foot massage from her not-so-secret young surfer boyfriend.

I went over to the door and rapped on the wooden panel below the flywire.

'Is that you, Pierre?' she said, in her sexy, smoky voice. She preferred the exotic appeal of the French version of my name.

I went in, a glimpse of a painting of her shapely arse on a large canvas, right in your face by the wood stove. She was sitting in semi-darkness at the kitchen table down the far end of the L-shaped room. I sat down on a gypsy chair opposite. Even in the low lamplight I could see she'd aged.

A bottle of champagne slid in my direction. 'Where have you been, Pierre? I've been expecting you for two whole nights.'

'I've been holed up in a place down on Horseshoe Bay. Trying to recover from a terrible year.'

She laughed. 'You haven't turned into a monk, have you?'

'I told you about it over the phone.'

'That didn't sound like *you,* Pierre!' – as if I'd confided nothing more than discovering a bald patch.

'Everything leads to cancer,' she said.

'Don't go there,' I retorted. 'For men it's a case of "damned if you do, damned if you don't".'

'Too much thinking was never any good for you,' she said, getting up and rummaging through a stack of CDs and eventually choosing obscure World Music. To keep the conversation going more than anything else, I asked why she hadn't been at open mic.

'I don't go there anymore,' she said. 'They're a lot of boring old farts. It's nothing like when you and the blues guys were around. The good old days.'

She filled our glasses with more bubbly and cranked up the music. 'These days it's a party for one down here. Now I know how you must've felt, Pierre. I was in a relationship with a gorgeous man but he turned out to be a bastard. I've never been so hurt by a man before.' Being potent hadn't stopped me suffering at her hands after we broke up. I'd gone overseas to escape her but she'd send cards and even ring me, when I was virtually untraceable. Over that year spent in New Zealand, I'd remained reluctantly celibate. Now, while unexpectedly back at the beloved kitchen table, I thought back to a weekend around the time of our split-up when I'd used the element of surprise, knowing she'd be away and the key would still be under the flowerpot. It was around the time I'd been having a recurring dream about this gorgeous old house. In the dream it was more like a film set than the actual house she'd once said I could be part owner of 'if I played my cards right'. In the dream, her six-year-old son was in the shadow of a tree in the front yard. I walked the gauntlet of film-star types. She was waiting for me in her leopard-skin mini at the end of the line. In real life she didn't come back from the post-bust-up holiday and I slept alone in our old bed, masturbated myself to sleep and missed her terribly all Sunday long. Then, after mending her front gate with wire, Balinese motorbike style, I drove back to Adelaide and my bolthole. I knew it was goodbye to the rambling old mansion by the sea, even though it had entered my blood.

She returned from the bathroom and offered me a rollie. After six months not smoking, I suddenly felt like one. I lit up and watched the smoke curl into the air and mingle with her perfect smoke rings. She regaled me with more tales of the bastard boyfriend.

I pretended to listen. Maybe everything would transform back into the golden era just by forgetting about cancer. Her gypsy-like quality seemed to hold the secret, the promise of impossible things. Her presence alone brought the unknown back into the equation. The endless stories about the bastard only made the here-and-now seem more possible.

After coming round to fill up my glass she stumbled, steadied herself with a hand on my shoulder, and draped herself round my neck. Our lips met in a clumsy, brief kiss, and there was the old familiar scent of the wild black hair and a millisecond of phantom power in my groin. She retreated to her chair, putting the table safely back between us.

I got up and found a CD I'd completely forgotten about. I'd posted it to her on a whim, a recording of four songs with my mate in Sydney. But hearing it only reminded me of the days when I'd been my former sexual self. Before the first track had even finished she got up and hit the stop button. She told me my music was boring and put John Lee Hooker on instead.

I couldn't really argue with John Lee – even if her lack of tact hurt. It reminded me why we'd split up.

I suppressed a flash of anger with another glass of red wine – the champagne having disappeared long ago, and let John Lee's bottleneck blues do the job. I left soon after, before the night could get any murkier.

We kissed air-guitar-style cheek to cheek at the back door. I walked off across the lawn, feeling free to be out of the old house, thinking not of what I'd missed out on but what lay ahead with Anna. I was closing the unconscious door as well as the actual gate to her arcane garden when she called out, 'Everything leads to cancer!'

I was happy to give her the benefit of the doubt. She was probably only trying to help me put my demons in perspective.

6

I woke early and made up my mind to go for a swim. My penis felt swollen. But it was only wishful thinking. It was the new undies clinging like Glad Wrap, without the glad. I lay there feeling myself, fantasising, and managed a bit of swelling but not much more. The surgeon's words of advice encouraged me to go on: use it or lose it. I got up and went to the toilet. Magpies were greeting the dawn, gargling up in the pines at the back of the flats. I suddenly missed our cat, the way she'd rub against my leg in the morning when I stood at the toilet bowl. A former street cat, she was a true survivor with plenty of lives still left. When I was recuperating in bed at home after the operation, she would lie on my wound, purring. She knew where the weak spot was and never came close to clawing the catheter bag.

Walking through Memorial Gardens after the swim, houses started to take shape in a dawn mist hovering over the bay. The last time I'd been up and about this early had been on the morning of the operation. We'd driven to the hospital on the cusp of night and day, an ethereal world that reflected my insubstantiality.

***

Not speaking. Driving to our fate along ghostly grey streets at the ghastly hour of 5.30am, preparing for dire times when I felt most vulnerable.

Anna parked in the all-day car park. She was there for the long haul. Ever since the pre-admission tests and consultations I'd been on an irreversible treadmill, but not really believing the allotted date would finally happen.

We sat in a terrible holding area. I had my travel bag at my feet, this time not bound for overseas or the bush. Everyone in the waiting room had a bag. No one looked at anyone else. There was hardly a word spoken as we pretended to read magazines and newspapers. All pretence. Yellow light filtered in through antiseptic white curtains from the day outside, which seemed to mock those assigned this dreary room. I sensed the stoicism, and the potential for a stampede. I for one felt ready to flee the silence of the lambs.

My name was called.

At the counter, I glanced back at Anna, who immediately joined me. I could tell she was struggling when we kissed. 'I'll be waiting for you,' she whispered.

My old self disappeared as I was taken into a labyrinthine world of grey linoleum corridors and finally, a cell-like room. I was issued white fatigues

I had to tie from behind, made to feel helpless from the start.

On a gurney to a lift I wondered why I was being wheeled when I could have easily walked. The orderly cracked jokes as we went up through a series of gigantic lifts to yet another holding area. I was shovelled onto a bed in a room of empty beds. I thought about running away after a nurse peeled back the covers and left me.

I propped half in, half out of bed, and thought about the stats that applied to my age and test results: a fifty per cent survival rate of five years *without* the operation. At that stage I didn't even know whether our surgeon of choice would actually be on the other side of the heavy industrial-plastic, concertinaed doors at the other end of the room. On pre-admissions day, I'd been horrified to read the fine print at the foot of the page I had to sign. Patients without private health cover must agree to the possibility of not getting the surgeon of their choice. It sounded to me as if you could end up with a comparative novice; so I made what I imagined to be a radical request and demanded the clause be crossed out before I would sign the document. It all left me with the feeling that men's sexuality is rated as no more than a footnote in the great scheme of things.

The anaesthetist finally came and wheeled me through to a small room, the last port of call before the place of knives and bright lights. I desperately needed to know if our surgeon of choice was in the house. I was close to tears when I asked to see him.

The sandman disappeared, and next moment there was the handsome face of the man who held my destiny in his hands, eyes sparkling as he asked how I was.

Seeing him was all I needed. Then he vanished just as suddenly as he'd appeared. I saw my last chance to confess to his sidekick. The final card I could play, as he dabbed my arm with an alcohol swab.

'There's something I didn't mention on the pre-admission's day. My father had a throat constriction. It was the reason he didn't survive his bowel cancer operation. Because they couldn't knock him out, they had to use a local anaesthetic, so they missed a bit of the cancer. He had to have a second operation and it was too much for him. I didn't mention it on the pre-admission form.'

'Don't worry,' my knight in shining armour assured me. 'That was eighteen years ago. The technology's come a long way since then.'

That's when the sandman tricked me. He'd given me a jab that I assumed was to relax me. Pethidine sprang to mind. But it was the real thing. He'd sensed I was capable of doing an eleventh-hour runner, and his sleight of hand was the first thing I remembered upon waking up a new man.

***

It was the last day in my cocoon and Christmas was a butterfly wing's disturbance away. In the post-operation phone calls I'd had with siblings about this recuperative holiday, they sounded as if everything was back to normal just because I was out of hospital.

I cleaned up. Washed dishes, wiped surfaces, stacked crockery, and put the cane lounge back in its former position near the television. Then I stood at the kitchen window one last time, staring at some washing hanging limply on the line. A crow croaked farewell and so I croaked back.

During last checks, I found a radio on a ledge behind a curtain and tuned in to a talkback show, inviting listeners to share their Christmas shopping experiences. I sat down at the table and listened. It was the first time in a while that I'd laughed out loud. The final caller spoke about how the obscene amounts of food consumed at this time of year could feed the starving millions in India. Although laughing at some of the stories reminded me that I hadn't lost the physiological reflex of laughter, the final caller's sentiments only succeeded in bringing into sharp relief the nature of an erectionless future. Ever since the operation I'd experienced negative thoughts in an *absolute* rather than a *relative* way. Then *Silent Night* took me back to the magic of Christmas when I was a child. Buying presents for my army of relatives using the money I won at the Royal Adelaide Show for flower arranging – a fait accompli because I was the only entrant in the boys' section. It was a family tradition. My brothers before me had earned money that way to buy presents at Christmas.

The cleaners barged in bang on ten o'clock with enough cleaning paraphernalia to obliterate the slightest trace of my ever having been here. Not so much as a merry Christmas or a by your leave.

After lugging bags up the street, I turned in at Memorial Gardens and went to ground on a bench overlooking the bay. Tired from lack of sleep, I lay down and started to experience hallucinatory daydreams. A group of holidaymakers passed by and a little girl asked her mother why the man was asleep – to which there was no obvious reply.

The next bus to the city wasn't until mid-afternoon. I had baggage in tow. Even in this relatively innocent neck of the woods you couldn't risk leaving stuff unattended on the beach and going in for a swim. It was the first question I asked my surgeon at the post-operative consultation. When could I get back in the pool? Almost guilty about asking so soon after the catheter had been taken out.

I listened to the gulls down on the beach and daydreamed about the times I'd made love in the ocean.

The first time was with my first ever girlfriend, a tomboy to boot. We'd swum to the reef and back at Port Noarlunga, and did it in waist deep emerald-green water; next with a girlfriend at a beach on the

Mornington Peninsula, on the green moss of a rock pool. There was also 'the indoor swimming pool incident' in Melbourne, when I got an erection and to my dismay two policemen had entered, poolside, though it turned out they were looking for a locker-room thief rather than a pervert.

I lay there looking up through the umbrella-rib branches of a pine tree, worrying about going to my young sister's house in Adelaide and my brother's on the West Coast, and my future with Anna. Not long after the biopsy result a drunken woman bailed me up outside our local pub and for whatever bizarre reason said, 'You're obviously a virile man.' I walked on, aware of a crumpled-looking older chap smoking in the shadows reminding me of how I might finish up.

I eventually rose from the bench and hauled my bags in the direction of the post office. The same man who only a few days ago had welcomed me with open arms now bristled with resentment when I asked if I could leave my bags there for a few hours. Just the look on his face answered the question. I'd brought down the tone of the place. Though no other customer was present, I felt guilty about not having a hire car. I tried my best to make light of it, backed off and retreated to the Top Pub where, as if by magic, the good old publican appeared out of nowhere. It had been years since I'd seen Dino. I'd assumed he'd moved on. And he quite happily let me leave my bags in the cleaners' room, almost as if he'd been expecting me.

Gulls were wheeling over the beach as I walked the cliff-top path for a last look at Sugar Plum Island. Lines of swell all the way down the coast were obscured in a shroud of sea mist from an afternoon onshore breeze. This time I was determined to get out amongst the waves, even though the surf looked messy. I made my way down to the beach along the old path now overgrown with saltbush, and found my spot, a hollow porous rock akin to a tiny cave. At the height of summer this beach would turn into a splash of colourful umbrellas in otherworldly, blue light. Then, from dreaming on a towel, straight out into the action, diving under powerful surging waves that would test any weakness in the dental department. I still use 'Knights', the dead whale beach's official name, as my mantra for the cold blast to finish off the daily morning shower; a jump in the Great Southern Ocean's pure cold water.

I stared at the sea, aware of being the watched as much as the watcher. I thought of Anna's mindfulness training CDs and a technique for letting go of stress. Not seeing thoughts as the truth, just things that come and then pass away again. The training was said to be 'a glide path into meditation, a common sense wisdom' and the direct opposite of Western knowledge based on rational thought as the be-all-end-all. The gulls gliding at the edge of the water reminded me of the first time I'd brought Anna down here. Running around the beach with a film camera, using a high shutter speed to capture the fleeting patterns of birds' wings over sand.

I thought about my mum's affinity with the sea. She'd always maintained that the ocean helped her whenever she was trying to solve family problems. Just before coming on my pilgrimage I'd suddenly asked Anna to accompany me. But she reminded me about my craving for solitude. I felt like ringing her. I would've been quite content to re-book the flight there and then and fly back. Give seeing my siblings a miss. Not that I wasn't looking forward to going up and staying with my sister, which these days was as close as it got to replacing the sleep-out at Mum's.

My reverie was broken when voices drifted up from the other end of the beach. A boy and a girl were at the water's edge, throwing a red frisbee. I stayed out of sight until they disappeared up the new council stairs.

I had the place to myself again. The sky was an apple green and the wind was dying, so the swell was beginning to hollow out. I changed into my bathers, grabbed the flippers and jogged down to the edge of the water to test my body for the first time since the operation. Here at Knights Beach anything could happen, including drowning; I had no idea what lay ahead for a man facing my future. William James wrote: 'All action is thus re-action upon the outer world ... The current of life, which runs in at our eyes or ears is meant to run out at our hands, feet or lips.' I set my toes in the sand and wrestled with flippers under an indifferent sky. Only the seagulls bore witness as I edged out through powerful white water over submerged rocks, somehow remembering their positions like the back of my hand. And then I was on my way with no thought of stitches bursting, or pissing in public; nothing. I was in oceanic forgetfulness, exhilarated by action. A paranoid shark thought came and went.

I caught a wave shaped from the swell rebounding off the headland and the backwash from the rip, a bowl for a radical take-off. The wave took me all the way across the tiny cove and spat me out in the shallows. On the last day of my pilgrimage I felt almost back in my skin again.

7

I woke early, on a single mattress on the floor of my sister's spare room and remembered arriving by taxi to a house in darkness. Morning light was coming in through silk curtains. My watch on a polished wood floor made it six am.

I checked my jocks. The sanitary pad was dry but I needed to go to the toilet. I crept down the hallway and gave the door a nudge, expecting to feel the weight of the dog on the other side. Then I remembered. Their beloved god-spelt-backwards was dead. Darkness at first as I opened the hallway door, then pale lemon light fell on a framed photograph of our parents, up on the shelf above the lounge-room's potbelly.

Out the back of the cottage the heat of the day was palpable, straight in through the weatherboard. The same intense morning heat I'd experienced waking up at Mum's as a kid, and later as the prodigal son on unannounced interstate visits.

I stood at the toilet bowl looking out the window. Mottled garden shapes beyond the frosted leadlight window. The pink and yellow glass glowing in hues only an Adelaide summer morning could conjure.

I went back to bed in the cooler part of the house with a second-hand Somerset Maugham novel I'd bought in Port Elliot the day before while waiting for the bus. I put a blanket up over the silk fabric and found a desk lamp and started reading from where I'd left off last night, after struggling to get to sleep in the stifling heat. Even though my sister had chosen a beautiful beach suburb, the air was as still as the gulf water.

The sound of her MG sports woke me the second time as she reversed down the drive. It faded around a corner and was replaced by the cooing of pigeons in the eaves. A familiar sound associated with my parents' sleep-out, and also a particular walk back from Sunday school in afternoon streets lined with pepper trees. A silk scarf hung in the doorway, a symbolic separation of spare room from hallway when I needed something closer to a bunker.

I got up and had a quick shower while I had the place to myself, knowing my brother-in-law would already have gone to work. I felt grateful for his quiet exit, at some ungodly hour or other.

While I brewed coffee and unpacked I had a quick look at my sister's books in an alcove next to the unused open fireplace. There was a mixture of art and craft, and spiritualism and tarot. They made just enough money to pay the bills from her tarot readings and yoga classes, the rent from a couple of flats they'd invested in, and his work as a skilled labourer. And quite rightly were proud of now owning the place outright, even if a major means to that end – her career as a high school teacher, nearly killed her.

Over the phone a month ago she'd sounded as though my being out of hospital meant everything was back to normal, or at least that's what my feverish imagination read into it. Although it could equally have been that I was on the horns of a dilemma: wanting people to ask how I was and not wanting to talk about it at all.

I sat in sun at the tiny wrought-iron table in the courtyard with a coffee, a notepad, and the postcard for Anna I'd bought down the coast. I was about to start writing something I knew would probably turn into a love letter, when a blue A4 sheet fell from the stationery onto the brick patio. Unsolicited bulletins from the hospital inviting me to come to prostate cancer meetings started arriving in the letterbox from the day I left hospital.

I was now on their list.

I had been invited to nominate my poison from all the possible nametags: RP (Radical Prostatectomy), EBRT (External Beam Radiotherapy), BT (Brachytherapy), ED (Erectile Dysfunction), HT (Hormone Therapy), CT (Chemo Therapy), WW (Watchful Waiting), 'Other'.

I understood enlisting PC people to congregate could have benefits, but in my case it seemed a bit premature. I still didn't know if I was an 'ED' or an

'Other', and I wasn't quite ready to be defined as someone on the cancer 'journey'.

The appearance of the unsolicited mail on my sister's brickwork, took away the impulse to write. The courtyard was shaded by the neighbour's overhanging tree but I chose to stay in the soul-affirming sun. Mum's old pink cane chair sat in state in a shaded corner after living in her fernery for years. But its out-of-place presence here only highlighted an overwhelming sense of absence in general.

After a second coffee I started to relax. I felt more a part of my sister's wild garden. Succulents huddled around the table like silent wood spirits and I was transported back to the Monet exhibition in Sydney. Anna had suggested we go there to try and offset the shock of the biopsy results.

After Monet's impressionistic miracles we'd gone to the café for cakes and coffee, looking out over the water to gunmetal-grey battleships moored in the background. I felt a terrible pang of missing her. This pilgrimage was ill conceived. I looked over to Mum's chair for an answer but there was just deathly silence.

My sister asked me a 'big question' when she was about ten: What did I think of Christianity? I replied that you have to love yourself before you can love anyone else. She recalled a desk strewn with impressive-looking university books, when going away to ponder the answer.

Only the sound of her car coming down the driveway at the side of the house saved me from spiralling into the void. She got out and fetched shopping from the back, and before I had time to offer assistance was striding towards me. We hugged awkwardly with the shopping between us, and I helped her inside with the bags. She put on the kettle and stowed the shopping things away while I took a seat at their tiny kitchen table.

'I see you've remembered how to operate our nifty little coffee percolator,' she said, rinsing out in the sink.

'Isn't it time you got something a bit bigger for entertaining, as they say?'

'We don't really need bigger,' she said.

True. They'd become an island unto themselves and in that knowledge I felt less alone.

She poured the tea and started telling me her plans to renovate the kitchen and bathroom. She also spoke of her 'design for life'. She told me she planned to live to a hundred. I couldn't say much to that. Her design for the future left little room for the lost soul who was not ready to hear about longevity. By the time she'd finished swamping me in her designs the issue of my operation was conspicuous by its absence.

She got up and went over to the kitchen window. 'A pair of swallows usually perch up there on the trellis in the morning. That's Mum and Dad keeping an eye over me.'

I went and stood next to her. The whole yard was a shimmering mirage in the heat.

'Did I tell you I saw a bird fly past the hospital window when she passed?'

'Yes you did.'

'Big sis' saw it too. Did she tell you?'

Our oldest sister had been the first to leave the family. She married a New Zealand mathematics professor at the age of twenty-two and brought up a family in Wellington.

Yes,' I said. 'She did tell me about the bird flying past the window at the moment Mum died. In a letter I think. So you're not on your own with that theory.'

'It's not a theory. We're related to a bird clan.'

I let it go through to the keeper. The Christian faith I'd grown up in was firmly based on the resurrection as miraculous fact. My secular faith extended only as far as the values my parents had handed down. I knew they were gone forever, as far as anyone can say they know anything.

It didn't seem that believing one thing or another was the point. I would have been happy to be related to birds if that would bring back my erections. I did believe in a spiritual dimension to sex. The phallus was not just a mechanical means to an end, be it baby or orgasm. Although I knew nothing could be discounted about anything because no one *really* knew, at least science had always been about asking questions and then trying to prove theories from hypotheses. In other times I might have discussed her folksy beliefs and maybe agreed to disagree, or unearthed some commonalities. But I was now only painfully aware of having tunnel vision about what had happened medically. I simply wanted to hide under the table like a kid until my grownup kid sister went away. Then for some strange reason, Nina Simone's black voice floated up out of the void singing 'Feeling Good', birds up in the sky, the way they make you feel.

I felt that I had let my host down by getting cancer. I was too raw. I had to suffer in silence under her roof. I'd given her *Light On Yoga,* light years ago. And it was still there on her bookshelves. The mistakes I'd made in my youth, the rebellious acts of an idealistic young man outraged by the Vietnam War et cetera et cetera she'd misinterpreted as acts of heroism. My younger sister still believed in a vaguely hippie philosophy mixed with a fierce will to stamp her own sense of identity on the family tree. She had learnt about mortgages and investing, interest rates and negative gearing. Things I'd never been able to get my head around. She also planned to take her silk-screen painting talents up north one day, and exploit the lucrative tourist markets rather than, as I had, attempt to create a hippie utopia there.

I was aware of being a wraithlike spirit in her kitchen, mired in a mask. She was the one I had once taken around the neighbourhood in a pusher to show-off the tricks I'd taught her. But now I was no longer myself, and despairing that she hadn't divined my wounded pride.

In our lounge room at the age of sixteen, when my sister was barely out of nappies, I had listened to LP records on the new record-player our parents had bought, mainly for me. It was during my first year at university, all our other siblings had left home. Religious light through lace curtains in the living room in late afternoon fell on the record-player's honey teak top, which slid open on golden hinges. My Dylan, Donovan, Nina Simone, and Peter Paul & Mary LPs were beyond their command. I'd relegated their rarely played Mario Lanzas, sacred music, and *South Pacific* to the back of the pile.

I was no longer sure whether to address my sister by the name she had suddenly decided she preferred – the reappearance of the birth name that reflected a desire to be recognised as an independent adult I suppose, or the nickname the family had always lovingly used. I admired her youthful spirit and her exercise and dietary disciplines that made her look at least ten years younger than she was. But right now I only sensed our differences and, like John Lennon singing on 'God', I no longer believed in Zimmerman or Buddha or tarot or I Ching or Beatles or Jesus or Gita.

But she was on a roll telling me about financial matters that didn't interest me in the least, though I respected the sophisticated fiscal concepts. As she was outlining her financial blueprint, I was in a fog of war, trying to think of illness as metaphor, learning from my fate.

Then I rallied, and tried to be stoic as she showed me our uncle's paintings as well as her own rather good watercolour landscapes. But I wasn't really present. I was a statistical observer, from an outlier's provenance. It had felt awkward from the word go, from the arrival in the taxi to no porch light left on, a lingering sense of my late arrival being taken as a lack of respect.

***

After the trip to the city, I'd caught a taxi to an old school friend's and although the thought crossed my mind to ring my sister to say I'd be later than planned, I hadn't. I felt as though I was out of prison, having fun in the outside world. I was reliving old school memories, out of my skin for a moment in spite of having spilt the beans to my old mate and his wife. They were initially shocked but allowed me the space to 'confess and forget'. I suppose I'd assumed, under the circumstances, that family would intuitively cut me some slack about irrelevant things such as not being exactly on time. Sex was the most important thing. It had become crystal clear to me, with the unalterable wisdom of hindsight. But at least the jury on that issue was out for another eighteen months, by which time my natural erections would either have returned, or not.

I would have been better off in a motel than the spare room at my sister's. We were in the same trap. She wanted her old Superman brother back. I wanted Mum's old sleep-out. It was where I'd always gone to ground when the chips were down. She took me outside again and showed me round her garden. In the middle of a patch of bulbs was a relic that used to be in our older sister's first house in New Zealand. A blue and white porcelain coffee grinder with a small wooden box now packed with seedlings rather than coffee grounds. She told me the bulbs had been bought on a final outing to a nursery with Mum. Although most of the botanical information went in one ear and out the other, I enjoyed hearing about Mum's inner sanctum of old ladies telling my sister to get *this* Apricot Nectar rose and *that* Canna Lily. We wandered over to their new outdoor table under the flowering fig, which our brother, Doug, had built. A masterpiece in jarrah, the hardest of hardwoods, its circular design and dark timber reflected his down-to-earth spirit. I ran my hand over the perfectly crafted dovetail joints, a legacy of our old man's engineering perfectionism. I also happened to know the table was a peace offering after he told her what he thought of tarot. She wrote a letter in response. Stood up to him, which I admired. But I also admired his response in wood rather than words.

'He's done a great job,' I said.

She smiled. 'Yes, he has hasn't he? He's going to bring a drill over to make a hole for the umbrella when he comes to pick you up. When is that by the way?'

'I haven't decided. Christmas is still five days away.'

I felt like putting off anything that could be put off. All I wanted was *not* to plan. Preferably to just disappear off the map. Escape the medical memory of the last nine months.

She suggested breakfast out there at our brother's table and insisted on no help and went off to make it happen. As I sat under the flowering fig, I recalled the café overlooking the hospital grounds the first day I was untethered from the trolley of intravenous tubes. An orderly had been sunning himself on a bench in a clump of bamboo, the smoke from his cigarette spiralling up through the cane the only hint of a private life. The next day, after moving my bowels for the first time since the op, I was cleared to go home. Kissing the *Be A Man* sign goodbye, then walking under the old turn-of-the-century archway and out through the gate in the low brick wall where the smokers sat. Finally back out on the street. Waiting at the taxi rank on cloud nine. Feeling that it was actually better to take those first steps without Anna, who had been unable to get time off from work to pick me up.

My sister set down the tray of breakfast things. I helped her unload muesli, milk, yoghurt, a bowl of fruit, and the tea.

She hoed into the cereal and asked if I'd spoken to my fellow prostate cancer brother.

'Not much,' I said. 'I feel bad about that because he was the only one I could turn to after my biopsy result. His advice to take it one step at a time was manna from heaven when I was drowning in a sea of medico information overload.'

She poured the tea. 'When I spoke to him after his operation, he said "life's a lottery". And now I almost forget he's ever *had* cancer the zero air space he gives it.'

I considered how to respond.

A few years ago she had to give up school teaching due to stress, having been diagnosed with a medical condition that was serious but not life-threatening if treated. When her symptoms reached a critical point it was lucky that our older sister happened to be visiting from New Zealand, and knew there was a drug that could 'cure' it. My sister had reluctantly agreed to be taken by ambulance to hospital. Down the track, years later, she told me she had only needed to take the medicine for a couple of months because she apparently cured herself with yoga.

I looked her directly in the eye.

'His PSA was very low. Mine was through the fucking roof. After the operation the surgeon said I would probably need help. Meaning, injecting my dick to get an erection, maybe for the rest of my life.'

There. It was finally out.

'I must say I was surprised when you rang to say you were coming over. It would've taken me the best part of a year to even *contemplate* stepping out of the house after having my temple messed with like that.'

I regretted telling her. She flicked her long hair and continued. 'I reckon we can heal ourselves through imaging.'

'Through what?'

'Projecting life-affirming images to the area instead of dwelling on the damage. I'll certainly be putting my psychic energy into healing your nerves.' She stood and collected the breakfast things and headed back to the house. A couple of willy-wagtails were flitting about in the fig tree after the Mad Hatter's tea party. I stared at tea-leaves at the bottom of my cup then refocused on my brother's carpentry, which still seemed gift-wrapped in his gritty spirit.

I received a card from him not long after getting home from hospital. 'You're coming good by the day. The iron man arises.' It was a reference to an old football adage he'd instilled in me as a boy – turning into *an iron man* in the face of his bullet-like football passes, which stood me in good stead when I eventually played Australian Rules football in Sturt's senior side, when the boyhood dream to play in the big league became a reality.

Sitting at his table in the claustrophobic forest that her garden had turned into, I realised how little either of them understood my medical situation. How naïve even *his* loving words had been – as if my sexual future would be solved in willing an ironclad mind into being. Let alone imaging a miracle.

It was now a dead hot Adelaide noontide. I heard my own voice give counsel: *Siblings remember you the way you were, not what you might become.*

I found myself daydreaming back to adolescence, sitting in a pew at the back of the Methodist church while my oldest sister practised pipe organ midweek. Witnessing adjustments to the coloured organ stops and then the enormous chords swelling forth, magical notes snaking up the varying lengths of rose-pink and golden pipes. Even as a boy her music had transported me.

***

I was doing the dishes when she breezed back in from a manic weeding mission in spite of the heat.

'Don't worry about the dishes,' she said. 'It'll only wake sleeping beauty.' Her husband had chosen the life of the healthy outdoors, which meant early to bed, early to rise. The weekends were his only sleep-in time so I took myself off to the lounge room and watched television with the sound on mute. White blobs gradually resolved into cricketers. Then a close-up of a cricket ball being rubbed up and down, up and down on a cream crotch stained red. Shining one side of the ball to get reverse swing later in the day, when Perth's famous Doctor blew in off the Indian Ocean. I watched in a trance as the cricket was intercut with Hitchcock's seagulls massing at backward square leg, the picnickers on the banks of the Swan blissfully unaware. My gaze drifted to the crocheted rug I was sitting on, a patchwork quilt that must have taken Mum months to finish. Her trademark light and dark greens, double blues and pastel yellows. The bedroom door opened and my brother-in-law appeared, rubbing sleep from his eyes.

'Good morning or is that afternoon? It's good to see you, brother. Sorry I missed your arrival last night. I was in bed by eight.' It immediately put my lateness into a bit of perspective.

We shook hands over the back of the couch and I apologised. Don't mention the war. A couple of years ago he wrote a line or two at the bottom of one of my sister's letters to me. He'd been recovering from an angle-grinder accident that nearly sliced his toe off.

'My toe has now made a full recovery,' he wrote. 'And you were so right when you shared your experience about your old back injury. How being laid up forces you to see things differently.'

He threw himself down on the couch by the window and turned the sound back on. But after watching for a while he was asleep, mouth wide open, as if recovering from jetlag. He claimed to love his outdoor work, but he was beginning to look older than her, even though he was the younger. He had once been a champion amateur wrestler, and was also naturally curious about the world and had a homespun philosophic bent. Despite still having a much fitter than average mid-forties male body, I did wonder how much longer it could hold up. Labouring was a young man's caper. I'd done some spells of labouring work myself over the years. It could be more than backbreaking.

By the time the players were walking off the field for lunch, I decided to head up to the guest room and have a siesta myself. I grabbed *The Goddess Within* from the bookcase and lay down on the mattress, opening to a chapter entitled 'The Moon'.

The moon was a female symbol that represented our unconscious desires and fears, including fear of losing control, but you must first enter a labyrinthine world of darkness before re-emerging into the light. Naïve art accompanying the text reminded me of the hippie drawings in a DIY manual, a back-to-the-earth manifesto about subsistence farming, including how to manufacture soap from charcoal and why to plant vegetables by moonlight. Then I came upon an idea plagiarised from the Stoics themselves: *There is nothing to fear but fear itself.* I read that I should *imagine floating in my feelings, back into the fluidity of the womb, to then emerge into the light.*

Dust motes filled the room in the afternoon light. It seemed much longer than a few days ago that I'd watched a sea eagle on a thermal, way up above the old crucifix-shaped wharf at Horseshoe Bay.

I dreamt I was in the childhood holiday place on the Mornington Peninsula, on the bottom bunk in a sun-filled room. It was quiet and peaceful, the sea faint in the background. Then the dream shifted to a dirt road near Wiseman's Ferry, in Sydney, where Jack our late kelpie was waiting for me at the wharf.

***

My sister and I walked to the beach along a wide empty street. The late afternoon light was hypnotic, intensely white, suffocating. Houses along the way bore no sign of life. I wondered whether going to the beach wasn't a sign of desperation on her part. The forlorn hope that the beach would somehow reunite us. I had fond memories of driving her to the sea after the traditional family Christmas lunch at Mum's and bodysurfing. We always got back in time for a Christmas tea of cold meat leftovers and salads.

When I looked up from a clump of gnomes in a front garden, my sister had vanished. The sound of motorbikes floated on the air. When I caught up with her on the esplanade, a battalion of bikies cruised by, like Vietnam Vets on Anzac Day. An article in the *Prostate News* pamphlet had made the point that blokes should pay the same respect to their bodies by having regular PSA tests as they did to servicing their motorbikes.

As they roared past in pirate pigtails and Germanic helmets, I wondered whether the boys would be as swashbuckling *after* the bad news. Or whether macho ignorance is bliss wasn't the wiser option after all. Fly in the face of obsessive medical statistics and ride on. Die young rather than risk losing the status of short skirts riding pillion.

We crossed in their wake and, uncharacteristically, I heeded a sign on a sandhill protection barrier – an unconscious admission I was no longer a match for the bikies' dare-devil attitude to life. I'd become old and conservative because of what I'd let them do to me. I trudged the long way round and by the time I reached the top she was already on the beach making a beeline for the water.

The tide was out. A few kids were splashing about in the shallows and the beach was starting to cloud over.

She'd chosen a spot close to the water and had peeled down to her bathers by the time I arrived. She waited while I changed into my Speedos with a towel round my waist. Not a soul in swimming due to recent shark sightings. No one taking chances. Children mollycoddled in politically correct cotton wool. How long since I'd seen a kid climb a tree? The world was obsessed with avoiding risks. Although young men – and nowadays women – were still being sent to foreign countries to fight old men's wars.

We waded out past an artificial rock formation covered in lime-green carpet masquerading as sea moss. She plunged in and we swam off in opposite directions. After a few unsatisfactory attempts to simulate my lap swimming, I was back in the shallows watching children play King of The Castle. I got out of the tepid water and lay on my towel, staring at the sky and thinking about Knights Beach twenty-four hours ago. Once upon a time I would have been transported in this lemony late-afternoon light, happy to doze on the sand. Now it felt as if death had crept closer, holding my sister at arms-length from me.

After pretending to read, she suggested a walk to the jetty. At the edge of the water I scooped up handfuls of wet sand, as she walked off down the beach, her blonde hair haloed in the setting sun. I let sand slop back into the water and imagined her puzzling over why we had suddenly become strangers. I recalled the Big Question she'd put to me when she was a kid, about Christian love. And my response about loving yourself before you could love anyone else. She had wanted me to walk with her, into her astrological design for the future. The idea of the impossible was anathema to her. She wanted her former brother back. Not the sad stranger he'd become.

As I got closer, and against the civilised tenor of the beach, I yelled out: 'I had a dream about Jack the dog!'

She turned and stared.

We stood in the shallows, facing the sunset. I told her about our old dog waiting for me in the moonlight at Wiseman's Ferry.

'The moon symbolises a journey into the unknown,' she said.

'I think it's more about an incident Anna told me about,' and recounted how Anna let Jack off the leash as he sniffed around the open gate to his old place. In he went. After a few minutes he re-emerged, looking up at her as if to say 'Now I know my life is with you', and trotted off to our place two doors down.

We spent a quiet night watching television, while I thought about my sister's idea of the future becoming a journey into the unknown. Just before going to bed, I went out and stood under a moonlit sky in the courtyard and rang Anna. Her voice kept dropping out. I paced up and down trying to find a clear spot and walked into a spider's web.

After we'd hung up, I thought about her voice, how there had been something different in her tone. There had been no 'I miss you'. No thread that connected the past and the future.

I felt a frightening flash that I'd lost her.

***

I dressed next morning without showering. I was planning a walk to find a quiet café where I could sit and think on my own, when a fish lunch was announced for 12.30. So I tore down the heat-shimmering esplanade, scanning every side street for a sign of alfresco activity. In the end I settled for a hotel at the Grange. At least it was respite from the heat and there was an espresso machine and a waiter who delivered good coffee to my table under the awnings. I sat there staring at the gulf waters, unable to even read the paper. It occurred to me that you were expected to 'move on'. It was what was behind the hurt look on my sister's face when I'd risked letting my solitary walk take precedence over lunch.

On the way back I took a last-minute detour down the main drag to buy a hat. I was contemplating becoming a beret man like my father had when he retired. From mechanical engineer to avant-garde Frenchman overnight. It had been a trend amongst retirees, adopting the look of the archetypal Frenchman.

I came alive for a moment or two while trying on hats, engaging in banter with two women from Victoria as unprepared for the heatwave as I was. They became my mirror, my fellow wine-tasters as it were. They told me a hat suited. I knew they were lying. No hat ever suited. My head disappears inside hats of any persuasion. But the women insisted the fedora was made for me. In the end I acquiesced, overpowered by forgotten female pheromones. I hurried back feeling like a new man in my new hat.

I was a convert to retail therapy as I rushed towards the side gate, announcing my shopping triumph. 'Like my new hat?' I called out, the child in me returning home from school, yelling out the day's news before he'd even got in the gate. Knowing Mum would be at the kitchen sink by the tiny window that looked out onto the grapevine by the side of the house.

They were already at lunch under the fig, so I had to come down from my shopping high and adapt to the grown-up scenario confronting me. I sat and took off the hat and helped myself to the remaining fillet of fish and some salad. I'd brought the Sunday paper back and despite the cold reception, tried to interest them in an article about the demise of the Murray River mouth, an area my sister was familiar with.

They were nearly done. I felt like a schoolboy made to stand in the corner and not speak. They left me frozen in a dramatic flourish about the demise of the River Murray, the newspaper already tomorrow's fish and chip paper, dead on the ground. A few moments later my brother-in-law re-emerged from the house and headed to the shed. He cast a sheepish look my way as if to say: 'I feel awkward too, brother, but that's life.' And of course he was partly right. It was expecting too much of family to understand the pain. I began to wonder whether Anna hadn't been right in gently suggesting that I could always 'go and see someone'.

It had also been expecting too much of retail therapy to fix my head. I never saw the hat again. It vanished right off the holiday map after its flash-in-the-pan moment of glory on top of my obsolescent middle-aged skull.

First thing next morning I made a split-second decision to leave my sister's and go to Adelaide and find somewhere to stay. I would then ring my brother, and tell him where he could pick me up.

8

I walked to the train station. Soon, nondescript suburban backyards were blurring past. I regretted ever leaving the shores of the Great Southern Ocean, where double oxygen ozone molecules damp out negative thought waves. I comforted myself in the thought I'd soon be with 'old faithful', Doug. Religiously taking the kid brother to football games each weekend; passing on tips about the game. At least I'd been his faithful nail holder while building the huts and go-carts. His adopting me as his special brother probably helped compensate for having been cast as pig in the middle, wedged beneath two older brothers and a sister and baby brother who slept in the same bedroom. He had been like a second mother to me, demonstrative, caring, behaving in a way that was not typical of fathers in those days. Not that Dad wasn't a great father. He was. He used to ferry us around hither and thither, including taking me to the parklands for kick-to-kick with the footy, and was always ready to help with homework.

I entered the city of churches by stealth along subterranean arcades, and emerged into the heat of a deserted King William Street. Rundle Mall felt only a bit better. I walked past the giant silver balls where, back in the eighties, I met my daughter whenever I was over from Melbourne. The café in the East End had perfect incognito lighting. I ordered coffee and found a dark table down back near the toilet. From here I could keep an eye on the passing parade in Rundle Street. I didn't have a clue as to my next move. I pined for the solitude of The Dolphins. Instead, I sat there sipping coffee, worrying over my little sister. For all she knew I was suffering from 'no more than depression'.

But after two long blacks, I began to accept my solitary table. Being in the café started to feel like the height of civilisation compared with the void of my sister's. After feeling as if I were to blame, as if I'd let her down, that it was my fault I'd been diagnosed with prostate cancer, the panicky feelings gradually subsided. I hunkered down in the dark against the weather and the psychic heat. It had been as simple as the timing of yesterday's fish lunch that had caused it. I needed a long leash after all those appointments with the white coats. I felt like screaming from the void to anyone I'd lied to over the fucking phone, I was bloody well *not* fine.

I went out into the grey street to look for a table, and a stab of sun on my cheek seemed miraculous.

***

I did have a certain faith in miracles. I'd gone to see a Chinese herbalist the day I'd been diagnosed, and beyond. I'd always had more than a passing interest in traditional Chinese medicine. In the eighties, Chinese medicine helped me when Western medicine had not. Conversely medical science got the job done when alternative approaches took too damned long. The first time I saw the herbalist, Kevin Lu, I was freaked out of my mind. I asked him if he could get me out of trouble. But after looking at my PSA and biopsy results, he advised me straight up that I should have the operation. He told me he could help me before and after the operation, that I should see him on a regular basis for five years.

Two days after the operation the surgeon came to my bed smiling and told me he was very pleased with 'the margins' and that he had never experienced so little blood loss. I credited, without proof, the herbs I'd been taking for three months on a weekly basis. And thought of more nerves being spared due to less blood hindering my surgeon. Quite apart from helping ensure I would not become incontinent. He also said it had been 'a nasty one', which I had 'probably had for years'. He told me the operation had taken six hours and he had made sure I was his only patient on the day. While I had been unconscious all those hours, Anna was in the hospital café, reading and drinking coffee. He rang her the minute he finished and when I woke up smiling, with the realisation I'd survived, she was there, by my bed.

It was only as the surgeon was about to leave, poised at the gap in the white cyclorama drawn around my bed, that I plucked up the courage to ask in a low voice, aware of other ears in the very public ward: 'How do you think I'll go with ... you know?'

'You're probably going to need help,' he said. After his honest reply I stared up at the ceiling, mentally underlining *probably.*

***

Christmas shoppers were rushing about in Rundle Street but my sister's face kept floating back up. Her look of disappointment when I'd said I needed to have a long walk. I had not lived up to her expectations. I had failed to move on. I was no longer qualified to wear a superhero's outfit.

I was tempted to bum a fag off someone but knew it would be like a red rag to a bull. I'd given up for the operation so why succumb to a slow death from cigarettes after I've just sacrificed so much for a longer life? I still wished my sister-in-law had never rung me. After my third coffee I rang my sister. She either didn't pick up or wasn't home. I left a message: 'Sorry about the abrupt exit. And sorry for dumping my negative shit on you. Thanks for your hospitality. My bag is in the guest room ready to go. I'll ring Doug and let him know where to find me. Sorry I wasn't much of a guest. Love always. Your brother.'

I walked a couple of blocks to a hotel and was pleased to find the same octopus-green tiles and U-shaped bar that I remembered. Possibly even the same men and women hunkered over their beers. I circled the Exeter for a while. The smaller bar at the back was connected to the front bar by a small window that had always reminded me of the pantry at my grandmother's fabled place in Melbourne. There was also an anonymous atmosphere after the implosion at my sister's. I still couldn't settle, kept going round and round. As if by moving I would keep the thing at bay. It had settled on my shoulders like soot from a hospital's incinerator stacks. Eventually I came to ground in a blissfully empty lounge room, soft country music playing from speakers high on the wall. With a glass of cold white wine, I chose a table away from the street window and at last felt safe enough to sit down.

I decided to book a room in a motel not far from the old suburb. I rang the number and fortunately there'd been a cancellation. It was not the Ritz but it was affordable and in a quiet, tree-lined street. I was about to head out when I received a voice message from my sister saying she hadn't expected me to be a model guest. She just wanted to look after me, as Mum would have. She signed off with love, which made me feel all was not lost.

A bus took me down King William Street past the *Advertiser* newspaper building. I glimpsed the entrance to the cobblestone laneway leading to the car park where I was allowed to park my car in my teens because I was the chief mechanical engineer's son. The bus went round Victoria Square then headed through Colonel Light's park lands. I was finally able to breathe again as we travelled south along Unley Road into tribal heartlands. Landmarks flashed by.

The office block where I'd courted my first girlfriend, who'd written me a poem. I still remembered the line, 'his smile is like a child's dream'. It brought back being seventeen again, being with her. She was the first to call me Pierre, for all the right reasons. I craned my neck to see the junk shop where I'd bought the pink table for my bolthole, after the break-up with Zelda. The table that was now in Sydney under the window that looked out over Callan Park and the old lunatic asylum tower.

We passed the hotel where Sturt's captain had been publican in the sixties. It was now gentrified, almost beyond recognition. Then up ahead, Unley Oval itself, and Woolworths opposite, where, on a stage in the car park, I'd celebrated with my Sturt teammates the club's Golden Era Grand Final victories in front of hundreds of adoring fans.

After getting off the bus I stared into shop windows, then walked along Unley Road past James's Funeral Home, where I'd gone for my father's viewing. His death mask had reminded me of a Samurai warrior's, lips curled down in disdain at the very idea of surrender. I hadn't been able to go right up to the coffin. After that one glimpse, I swivelled on my heels on the polished cold linoleum floor, and fled to the safety of the car and waited for my younger sister.

I walked past Wattle Street where the first girl I dated had lived. If riding a girl home from school counts as dating. At the time it was the equivalent of conquering demons after nights of thinking about her and breathlessness in the morning at the prospect of seeing her wheel her bike into the schoolyard. Timing it so that it wouldn't be too obvious, desperate to actually say hello to the goddess.

The darkened doors of a mostly unchanged Cremorne Hotel, for some reason, brought to mind Robert Rose. I'd read *Rose Boys,* written by his brother Peter. His father had been coach of the Collingwood Football Club, no less, and Robert played Sheffield Shield cricket for Victoria and football with Collingwood. But then a terrible car accident in his twenties had left him quadriplegic. He is depicted as a man with an all-or-nothing attitude to life after the accident, refusing to be thought of as disabled. Staying out of the public eye, eschewing disabled parking spaces or competing as a wheelchair Olympian.

I turned off Unley Road near the girls' grammar school. Their below-the-knee pale-blue uniforms had signified studious rather than sexy to my innocent Methodist eyes. No wonder The Rolling Stones blew our minds. Down a side street I turned in at a stately hedge and walked down a gravel driveway beside an Edwardian pile. My old Unley High School mate had been a doctor for years. I played tennis with him at school and whenever I was back here at Christmas and at a loose end, I could get a game on his lawn court.

Around the back was the pride and joy, recently mown. The lines freshly painted white. The cocker spaniel barked and appeared when I knocked at the tradesman's entrance and then after smelling my hand, rolled over for a pat. No one was there. But the detour had brought me closer to my family home. It was peaceful off the main drag. I walked blocks without seeing a soul. It had been my father's route to work to miss the traffic. I wandered along a street until it reached a landmark where Brown Hill Creek flows under a bridge. Opposite was the first house my parents had lived in after their migration from Melbourne in the thirties. For a moment it felt as if I'd never existed.

I leant over the bridge. The creek was dry. Just grey river stones where yellow-brown water would flow, deep enough in the winter in certain places for my brother and I to entertain launching a raft and turning into Tom Sawyer and Huck Finn going down the Mississippi.

I spent another hour or so mooching around the old suburb and despite getting closer and closer to the old house, decided to leave it as a beautiful memory and get a taxi to my motel.

While waiting for my brother to collect me, I tried ringing Anna in Sydney. I only got my voice on the answering machine and hung up without leaving a message. After an unplanned night all to myself I was ready for my brother's company. The image in the mirror in the motel's bathroom after the shower hadn't been all that bad. I thought about a conversation I'd had with one of Anna's relatives about the pros and cons of the operation. Out of the blue he'd said: 'As a boy you never even missed sex. We spend a quarter of our lives *not* missing it.' I also thought about the surgeon's honest reply just after the biopsy, when I'd told him about the blood in a condom during the time of squirreling away sex before the hibernation after the deed had been done.

'That's because of what I did to you in the biopsy,' he said. You'd think alarm bells would've rung. Doug was not a holocaust denier but over the phone I'd had the impression he wouldn't want to hear about semen and blood, and then no semen. I wasn't sure how I would handle being with him again. Our relationship was still based on the early years. Building huts, making footy scrapbooks, playing outside until dark. Going to every suburban oval together to see our team get regularly slaughtered.

9

I threw my backpack into his four-wheel drive alongside a huge toolbox and the bag he'd picked up from our sister's. He drove to Woolworths when I mentioned that I wouldn't mind a new T-shirt and clip-on sunglasses. Being with him made even these little acts seem significant, as if it were a new beginning to innocence, a return to something that could transcend the shit that had hit the fan, the brotherly balm that would do the trick no professional could.

I felt at home as we drove out through the suburbs. We'd been so close that while riding bikes we would sometimes say the same thing, even after long periods of silence; as if we could read each other's mind. But then came the lost years when he was in the Murray Mallee, teaching off his Education Department bond while I was at university and playing league football and getting involved in anti-capitalist politics. For a decade we didn't communicate. Years later he would say: 'I always assumed you'd rejected me for being too *bourgeois.*' Then, after waking up alone in yet another communal household in Melbourne, I'd rung to say I was coming over to the shack for Christmas.

By the time we were north of the city, we'd covered familiar stories, including some I'd already heard from our sister. It was comforting to sit back and be driven by my surrogate mother and make small talk, forget about the troubles. Then, just as I was imagining the lovely drive ahead and having a cold beer at his local before the final stretch to the Ponderosa, he made an unannounced detour and drove into a new housing estate in one of those soulless outer northern suburbs. We stopped in front of a brick-veneer house.

'I'm just going to drop a Chrissie present off to Betty. She's an old friend who's had cancer.'

He jumped down and went and knocked on a door decorated in Christmas ivy and red berries. After knocking a few times, he left the package in her letterbox.

He was smiling when he hauled himself back up into the cabin. 'Two years ago Betty was told she only had six months to live. A palliative nurse arrived on the doorstep one day, expecting her to have her bags packed. Betty told her where she could go.'

My brother chuckled. 'Betty's as tough as they come. She'll only go on her own terms, no one else's.'

I stared out the window at nothing in particular as we drove back out to the freeway. There were shades of the iron man underlying the Betty story. It was only natural for him to assume I'd take it like a man, keep shtum and move on to rise again.

'What sort of cancer has Betty got?' I asked.

'Ovarian. But it wouldn't matter what it was.' He made a dismissive gesture. 'She'd handle it the same. She refuses to go down without a fight. I admire that sort of fortitude. From the Latin fortis.'

It dawned on me that the sidetrack to Betty's had been more than just killing two birds with the one stone. There was a parable lurking beneath. An example of the positive-thinking school of thought. My brother was on a roll.

'It's the same attitude you've always had,' he said. 'I remember when the Unley High School selectors were watching you play in a trial game for selection in the First Eighteen football team. When you were in Intermediate, only fifteen. I was walking behind them and happened to overhear one of them say "but he's too small". So I piped up: "He might be small but when he gets knocked flat he gets straight back up again."'

I kept gazing out the window. 'Yeah, I remember you telling me that.'

We passed the tidal mangrove beaches on the road north and then stopped at Port Wakefield for a toilet break. My brother seemed to know the subtext, incontinence, but made a joke about our oldest brother instead.

'At least JB doesn't have to worry about stopping for number one toilet breaks at the moment. With his poo-bag he can now drive the whole way over without stopping.'

Our oldest brother was still recovering from serious bowel cancer that required chemo as well as surgery. A month or so ago he'd told me they kept throwing up hoops and he just kept jumping through them. He had been the first to buy a shack on the peninsula and before building the new place had written a motto on the old wall. *Why Worry?* So his circus dog analogy felt like pure JB. Why worry indeed? He was the true iron man. Not that comparative thinking always worked on families.

The wheat silos of Ardrossan flashed by and, after a glimpse of the blue gulf, we drove inland. I began to feel the conversational void. He'd probably heard enough after having three brothers diagnosed with the Big C, suffering the guilt of the survivor. So I gazed at sparse bush and tried to free my mind. Tried to feel what he wanted me to feel. We were travelling through terrain similar to the Mid North, where my sporting brothers had played in tough country football associations. Both had been captains. Doug had played until he was forty. They had also both been deputy headmasters of primary schools. I'd seen one of Doug's recent end-of-year school photographs. He's sitting in his deputy's office in a straw hat with an ironic smile, his good-looking face hidden by dangling anti-fly corks, surrounded by adoring staff members.

I put on a CD Anna had given me for Christmas. Ryan Adams. I'd fallen in love with the soulful country sound wedded to his stream-of-consciousness storytelling style. It was difficult to hear the lyrics so I turned it up louder and hoped the driver wouldn't think I was still making some anti-bourgeois point. When I finally asked what he thought of the music, Doug said: 'I don't do lyrics.' It seemed a strange thing to say. As if he could be up front with me now. But I could not live without poetry in my life, least of all now. Maybe it was all in my imagination. People say things. It just wasn't his cup of tea and my perceived recent 'sickness' did not give me the right to override his taste in music. I'd forgotten. He didn't do music either. That was *my* sixties thing. He'd missed the Dylan inspiration by half a decade.

The voices in my head were endless. I was the spoilt little brother who had finally got his comeuppance. What my footy fanatic and overly proud brother called – even after I inexplicably walked out on the beloved game at the age of twenty-two – 'your independent rebellious spirit that was way ahead of its time'.

I hit the eject button and wound down the window and breathed in his far more real world. Eucalypts, manure, sheds, fields. A red harvester sparkled like a new matchbox toy in a far paddock. Then after rounding a long slow curve, flat, wheat-yellow paddocks and rusting farm equipment, sandstone ruins.

My brother fielded a call from his wife. He was wanted back in time for tea. So I knew my sentimental idea of beers at the pub had been scuttled. We turned down a dirt road but after a few dusty kilometres were back on bitumen. We passed the spot I'd stopped to take photographs a few years ago, when I'd driven Mum over for what would be her last trip. The strokes had taken more than her power of speech. She was just too damn old, too many things had broken down. And she didn't have Dad to ferry her around any more. At least our father had seen the fruits of my brother's labour, the transformation of a shack into a beach cottage. My brother's spirit was in the very grain of his Blue Horizon. In every joust and joint, in every enormous beam erected without his young brother around to hold a single nail.

We pulled into their enormous backyard and parked in front of the double garage. The doors were open, displaying the boat and caravan courtesy of his recent retirement package. I got out into blissful silence, into the purifying emptiness of an Edward Hopper painting.

I was shown to my room, the old master bedroom traditionally reserved for Mum and Dad, in the heart of the original cottage. I dumped my bags on the floor and noticed a cassette player thoughtfully provided, which nearly swayed me. I was being honoured with Mum and Dad's room but since my brother's extensions, it was a black hole in the morning. I prepared to become unpopular by asking for the spare room. I'd always stayed there in my pre-operation days so why not now? I'd be happy with the room on the other side of the house, in the new section. An office and guest room combined in one, there was morning light and an escape route to a small courtyard at the base of the derelict windmill. A ladder went halfway up, from where you could see the beach and the jetty and out over rooftops to the backblocks. I remember the Christmas my fellow cancer brother flew a box kite from the top of the windmill with an aerial attached for his ham radio because this spot was notorious for its weak signal.

There was a hint of disappointment in Doug's voice when I asked him about the other room. I had rejected what he thought was the honour of being given Mum and Dad's old room in the heart of the historic cottage. But it was one thing to imagine being close to siblings, quite another to suddenly be under their roof. My father had been opposed to my brother being with a married woman. I was on my brother's side, against him. I'd helped paint their secret house in the city when he brought her back with him from the bush and no one else in the family had known for months. He was a brother who'd always looked after me so, as a nineteen year old, I naturally supported him.

***

Next morning I was relieved to see a blue-sky day. I could get out of the house and walk for miles on my own. Maybe even find a new sense of self in the religious heat of Never-Never Land, the miles of sandhills stretching all the way to our oldest brother's shack.

My room looked out onto the front lawn. My brother had built a new picket fence and painted it pristine white. On the other side of the only strip of bitumen in town was a row of fibro houses, a glimpse of stubbled paddock out the back. I tried to get back to sleep but the voices and the breakfast sounds and the aroma of toast and coffee made it difficult. Eventually there was just a gull's cry.

I jumped out of bed, grabbed my towel and slipped out through the sliding door. I had a quick piss at the base of the windmill, then took the long way around the back of the caravan park to the headland. I exercised on the beach and then swam through crystalline water watched by fishermen on the jetty.

No one was around when I returned from the baptismal swim. I imagined they'd gone to do last-minute Christmas shopping and pick up the mail before everything closed for Christmas.

I brewed coffee and took a bowl of muesli out to the arbour. At the wrought-iron table by the old windmill I read yesterday's paper in a delicious backwater of green plants and creepers, a faint breeze off the saltbush.

A tractor rumbled past, a late-starter taking his fishing boat down to launch at the beach with no ramp. My brother had bought a cheap Massey Ferguson from a farmer friend and I knew he was looking forward to taking me out in his new speedboat.

The sound of shopping plunked down on the table in the long room that abutted the kitchen snapped me out of my reverie. My brother had built the Quinn Room in honour of the maternal side of the family, paying homage to Mum's father and also her brother, Uncle Arthur, a retired commercial artist. His portrait of our grandfather was the hero picture in the Quinn Room. Although our grandpa had been a humble house painter all his life, he had also been a very good artist. Some of his oil paintings, left to go to wrack and ruin in a shed in suburban Melbourne, were belatedly rescued and restored by my oldest sister. Our grandfather also cobbled together miniature works using bark and ink, depicting subjects such as an Aboriginal hunter throwing a boomerang at a kangaroo. When the rest of the tribe were at the beach, he would remain behind to fossick in the bush for materials. His son, Uncle Arthur, the retired commercial artist, once painted me a streetscape of where he though I lived in Carlton. It was a few streets out, but the scene brilliantly captured the character of the area. He once confided that James Quinn, our famous great-uncle, had the 'soul factor', which he himself lacked. After winning a travelling scholarship in Melbourne, to study in Paris, 'Jimmie' became one of Australia's official war artists during the First World War and remained in Paris and London most of his life. He has paintings, mostly portraits, in galleries in London, Paris, Melbourne, and in regional galleries such as Ballarat and Bendigo. Doug preferred our uncle's work over our famous great-uncle's because he related to the living man first, art second. The business of what constituted great art had no interest for him. In fact those arguments could get his hackles up. The Quinn Room was a wish fulfilment, a futile attempt to emulate the loaves-and-fishes tableau of our childhood summer holidays on the Mornington Peninsula. My brother's table mirrored our grandparents' table. Theirs, with its green linoleum surface, had to be long to accommodate the tribe of thirty each Christmas; my brother's honey-coloured masterpiece was built for a pride of lions that no longer existed.

The door slid open and he peered out into my improvised open-shade den.

'Had any breakfast yet?'

'I've had a bowl of muesli, thanks.'

'I've got the boat out of the shed ready to go. It's perfect weather for it.'

He disappeared back inside but left the sliding door open. I heard an impatient tone in his voice when he spoke to my sister-in-law. I was far away from thinking about recreational boating under a blue sky. Zooming around on water wouldn't do me much good.

Their voices eventually faded to another section of the house. The last dregs of coffee tasted good. The chirping of a bird comforted. I returned to writing the card that was turning into a letter too late to post to Anna.

'This place can't bring back my soul, my dear. And I'm truly sorry to say that. I have my mother's impatient nature and can't wait for the New Year to begin. See the surgeon. See you. My darling girl...'

A blue-tongue lizard crawled past my bare feet and disappeared into the succulents at the base of the windmill. I wanted to sit out there and let the saltbush wind whisper in my ear a little longer and think ahead to the real healing, between Anna and me.

When I finally emerged, they were sitting around the bottle-green glass table in the patio, with newspapers and cups of tea. I went to sit down. But Doug rose to his full height and said in a gruff voice: 'Let's not waste any more of the morning. I'll show you over the boat.'

The boat was up on the trailer connected to the Massey Ferguson. A huge outboard motor tilted up on the stern gleamed in the sun, the white hull's blue detailing matched the Blue Horizon theme of my brother's palace by the sea. He hopped up on the trailer and hauled himself on board. 'I'll run you through the basic safety protocol,' he said. I got up on the trailer and propping on my elbows looked at coils of rope, boating cupboards, oars, floats, and fishing rods as he began to teach me about PFDs, personal flotation devices.

I shut down.

It all floated in one ear and out the other. I'd come all this way to escape but even in the great outdoors there was no escape from bloody safety-first protocol. Why not just take her down to the water and head on out? I was in another word altogether, the world of Marianne Faithful's 'Lucy Jordan', driving her car at the age of forty-seven 'with the warm wind in her hair'. I'd had nine months of protocol to get me up onto the surgeon's table. I wanted no more protocol. I only understood *Broken English.*

I stepped down off the trailer: 'Sorry, Big Doug, I can't do this,' I said and walked back to the house, feeling disbelief boring into my back. Halfway across the bald lawn a three-cornered jack pierced my sole. I kept on walking. Refusing to limp.

The guest room suddenly felt horribly wrong. I was marooned. Surrounded by bleached-out streets ghosting in the heat. I went out to the arbour, and mercifully remembered Anna crouching on the brickwork there a decade ago, hunched over her sketchpad. When a crow finally broke the sullen silence, I began to see the boat incident in a different light.

At a deserted ocean surf beach on Phillip Island I'd stayed in my depth with a toe-hold in the sand while he swam out through huge waves and bodysurfed. There'd also been the recent event when he and a couple of mates nearly drowned after drifting out in a tinny while spotlighting for gar. A wave swamped them and the aluminium boat went to the bottom. They'd swum in the dark for hours against the current.

My brother was in the pantry stretching up to a cupboard using a library ladder, putting cans of food away. I was shocked to see he'd been crying. I focused on the tiny green-linoleum table lined with jars of preserved apricots, identical to Mum's, remembering the DVD in the show bag the hospital provided on the last day. An interview with a man who had been the alpha male of the family, who had finally accepted his new role as the eunuch and said he was 'a better man for it'.

My brother climbed down the ladder and stood on the other side of the table, squaring off.

I thought of the poster in the corridor of the hospital telling you to *Be A Man* and have the operation for the sake of your family. It was similar to an anti-conscription poster of the sixties of Uncle Sam in a top hat jabbing a long finger out at the viewer with the caption: *Your Country Needs You!*

'Sorry, Doug,' I said. 'I need lots of space at the moment. I can't handle organisation of any kind.'

He looked down, staring at the green linoleum as he hissed out: 'I just wanted to show you a few things you needed to know about the boat. It's too late now. The morning's gone. It's the best weather we've had for weeks. I thought *you'd* brought it with you. I've always missed having my young brother here with me.'

'Sorry,' I repeated, lame as a duck.

His face was taut when he looked up, fists still squared off on the table.

'Other blokes wake up in the morning, see blue sky and say, "It's a good day for fishing, let's go out." And then they do. But in my case it's like nothing's ever meant to work out. I'm always missing the boat for some reason. With your university-trained mind can you tell me why that is?'

There was a constricted tone to his voice, anger and vulnerability rolled into one, and a hint of Dickens' *Great Expectations.* I felt bad for having made this kind brother of mine look so *bereft.* As if his life hadn't been tough enough compared with my charmed existence, until now. I could not explain what had happened out there on the boat, under the sun. A flashback perhaps? I had no answer. His unintended boat pun only made me feel worse. The last three months had created a spiritual vacuum. It was more than just another blue-sky day to me. It was the end of the world.

He had no idea that being on my own in the morning had become an inexorable routine. He probably thought I was sequestering myself away just to be different, as usual, instead of being a normal guest and 'eating up all the good food' I was fed. 'It's *all* good food' father said after I'd told him 'you are what you eat'. It was all the fault of those bloody university professors. Abstract philosophy rather than real things made from wood. I was meant to sublimate my problem into boats, tennis, golf, and fry-ups.

It had been forgotten that I'd been their babysitter when they were living in their secret place with their child after he brought her down from the bush. It was Christmas '69. I'd given him The Hollies' record with 'He Ain't Heavy, He's My Brother' on the A side as a symbol of solidarity. The same year I'd first expressed my solidarity with the anti-Vietnam War protesters.

'We could still play tennis,' I said.

'That'll have to wait until it's cooler,' he said. 'We could play eight ball out in the shed if you like.'

His industrial-sized shed was divided into halves. Lathes and drilling machines down one end, pool table, bar fridge, and an old couch from Mum's down the other. Lining the walls were cards and postcards, including a number of my old personalised arty Christmas card collages, yellowing and curled up at the edges. On the wall near the pool table was a large map of Australia with coloured pins denoting all the places they'd been on their grey nomad trips.

The shed was surprisingly cool. Large skylights created the authentic pool-hall ambience I'd experienced with him in a semiprofessional hustlers' hall in the mid-sixties when I was about sixteen.

The double door at the back opened onto a patch of wild garden, and while he was racking up the balls I grabbed a stubby of beer from the bar fridge and propped in the sun half in half out of the shed. I took a piss on a patch of gravel by a hydrangea bush that was suffering from sunstroke and started to feel more relaxed out of the house.

He was methodically pocketing ball after ball, and telling me about an old mate of his who used to have a holiday shack here. He had visited recently. He had perplexed my brother by saying he couldn't understand why anyone would choose to actually *live* here after retirement.

'I told him it was all about relaxation. No traffic lights. No stop signs. What's hard to understand about that? Do you know what he said?'

I chalked up my cue after he'd finally missed. 'What?'

'Sounds boring to me.'

I could relate to the no traffic lights. But there was much more to it than that. Coming in through those wheat-yellow plains, I sensed what could only be termed a spiritual affinity with the place. You could disappear into the landscape.

The games continued.

I sat on the stool under the scoreboard he'd filched from an old codger. It had brass sliders and worn rosewood runners. A transistor radio was tuned to the only station with any sort of reception, playing Christmas carols. When I heard 'Oh Come All Ye Faithful' I half expected the old flatbed truck with the church choir to materialise in the street. The fellowship truck used to come and sing on Mum's corner every Christmas Eve and Mum would bustle forth with a tray of cordial and biscuits as Doug and I perched on the hedge for a better view. After they passed we jumped down and chased Christmas whiskers floating in their wake down the street on a balmy Christmas night.

The jetty was a shimmering silhouette, a golden black ingot. I was under the boardwalk because I'd let my brother down again. I'd offered to play tennis to make up for the boating disaster. Usually I would have thrived in the heat but before we'd even fired one shot in anger, I called it quits in a most uncharacteristic fashion. My heart just wasn't it because I couldn't stop thinking about losing my mojo. It was only by rebelling against sport that I could get through to him that I'd lost the desire to compete, and, as he knew only too well, there is no other way to play. It was a desperate attempt to show that the childhood iron man myth was just that. A myth. No *game* could sweep what had happened under the rug. My life had stopped. My emasculated form slumped down in the shade of the clubhouse, throwing in the towel in a very un-Dad-like way.

Miniature waves lapped at the base of the pylons. But at least the incognito darkness under the jetty was comforting after the intensity of the interrogative light up in the land of the living. A boogie board draped with a sodden beach towel drifted out between the pylons. I waded out and rescued it, but the beach looked mysteriously deserted. A middle-aged couple at a cement table under the barbecue shelter were drinking wine and watching the sun go down as I left the board outside the caravan park, and walked up to the house.

10

On Christmas night I found myself looking through boxes of university books stored here since the sale of our parents' house, four years ago. I was down on my knees looking at classics, when my sister-in-law called out they'd started the meal without me.

The books had escaped my father's great woodshed purge. It had been his way of getting rid of the side of me he'd never understood. But to be fair, he had waited years for me to come back and reclaim boxes that took up space in his shed. As a kid I'd loved the forty-four-gallon drum he used as a furnace for the Sunday burn-ups. As if flame and smoke belonged to the protestant Sabbath because the really sacred day was Saturday, football day. But the smell of hedge clippings burning on Sunday afternoons was hard to beat. Red flames licking around the bottom of an old rusted brown drum up on a few bricks for the fire to breathe.

I woke early and went to the beach. The sky was threatening rain. No one else was up on Christmas morning except a few kids on the jetty trying out new fishing rods from Santa. I did my mixture of yoga and isometrics on the beach and also the pelvic-floor exercises clenching buttock muscles together as if trying to restrain a fart while counting to ten. Then I swam a couple of uninspired pretend pool laps away from the jetty's holidaymakers. When I got back I brewed coffee and went out into the arbour. It was eerily quiet, apart from a solitary crow's descending black notes in a minor key. The air felt heavy and humid. The pale paddocks, the windmill, and the fernery combined to form the perfect bush curtain-raiser for Christmas Day.

He started singing 'Jerusalem': 'And did those feet in ancient time/Walk upon England's mountains green?' invoking the spirit of Christmas, trying to get me to forget the last five months. Have a bit of a laugh. But he was also stealing my thunder, my party trick from days of yore when I'd been full of confidence. My earliest association with the hymn was standing between Methodist pews, the rousing lyrics thundering over my head as the congregation – including my parents next to me – vented their emotion in the name of the Lord. Not knowing that an English composer in the middle of World War One had taken a poem by William Blake a century before, and turned it into a national battle song in Britain's darkest hours. During my university era, 'Jerusalem' became the socialist question: 'And was Jerusalem builded here/Among those dark satanic mills?'

Now the lyrics were more psychological than religious or political: 'Bring me my bow of burning gold!/Bring me my arrows of desire!/Bring me my spear! O clouds, unfold ... I will not cease from mental fight/Nor shall my sword sleep in my hand...'

Enter Freud and my troubles.

I would have preferred to stay out there, listening to the crow's black carolling or invoking Van Morrison's *Hymns to The Silence* rather than forming a brotherly duet *sans* piano. But I came to my senses and gave the deaf dog at my feet a pat and then went in to face the sudden silence.

We shook hands and wished each other merry Christmas. 'Give us a Christmas hug,' I said, ashamed of projecting my melancholia onto him. And he gave me a bear hug that squeezed any remaining bad vibes from the non-boating event right out of us. A year or so later he would describe himself as 'a pilgrim looking for a palliasse' when he flagged coming to Sydney to stay with us. His reference to straw bedding was the sort of thing only he would come up with. In our mid-teens we'd gone on a church camp together, to a beach south of Adelaide when palliasses were fashionable among all those, in the words of Leonard Cohen, 'Josephs looking for a manger'.

We spent the rest of Christmas morning holed up in the lounge room in the original cottage, resigned to the bad weather. Unfortunately it was not quite cold enough for lighting a wood fire, although that's precisely what I would have done with Anna.

My brother read snippets aloud from a book I'd given him for his birthday, a few months back: an autobiography by a former journalist who'd decided to leave Sydney and have a 'tree-change' on the south coast of NSW. While dubbing tracks from my old vinyl records to cassette, it felt as if the old days themselves were being re-recorded and we were on the same wavelength once again.

I was in the computer room writing up notes about Photoshop for a belated Christmas-cum-thank-you card for Doug when my oldest brother JB and his wife arrived.

They were all sitting around the circular glass table in the patio with a plate of biscuits and a fruitcake from the visitors. I'd always got along well with JB's wife. A school librarian for years, she was now on the brink of retirement and had the same macular degenerative eye condition as Anna's mum. After small talk about weather, and fishing, which JB was not doing much of these days due to his recent bowel cancer, he asked when I was planning to go back.

'Probably Tuesday,' I said. 'Maybe sooner.'

'You remind me of one of my grandsons,' my other sister-in-law, Doug's wife, cut in. So far we had managed not to rub each other up the wrong way. For some reason, she'd turned against me some years ago. I suspected it was to do with the unbreakable bond between me and Doug, and also resentment that no one ever gave him the credit he was due regarding *his* football career. She had once been a champion country tennis player, but a gammy knee now made playing impossible. But she knew her sport and, although she'd caught me off guard, I instinctively volleyed back.

'Like the wind? Unpredictable? Is that what you were going to say?'

'Something along those lines,' she said, with that wry smile of hers. The sentiment reflected what my father thought. I was a butterfly. But none of them now knew me from Adam, certainly not the scared, post-operation me.

To her credit she asked, 'How's your waterworks after the op?'

'Fine,' I said.

'Well you're all right then.' Case closed.

Once upon a time she had been as proud of me as my brother, or at least because of my brother. Maybe the boat upset had forced her to bury the hatchet. As I sat at the table, feeling on the outer, it struck me that JB seemed to smile a lot. I found that depressing. He'd jumped through all the medical hoops thrown at him. He was now almost out the other end of the cancer tunnel and I had to admit that his mental and physical toughness came as no surprise. He'd been reported for striking when he was captain coach of a country football team. As a kid I'd been shown the headline in the country newspaper: 'Captain Coach Runs Amok'. I knew what amok meant when I was fourteen, but it wasn't until years later that I realised *why* he'd run amok. An opposition player had said 'Did you forget your boomerang?' to an Aboriginal teammate of my brother's to try and put him off his game.

Whack.

The pathfinder of our family was before his time. Now he was dealing with chemo in a very Zen-like fashion, more confident than I'd ever seen him. It was as if he'd finally found voice at the age of seventy-three, even if an attitude rather than a literal voice. He seemed content to relinquish the fishing boat to his son, my nephew. Presumably because of the bowels, out in the deep-blue yonder. *Naturally,* I hadn't asked.

I felt like a cat on a hot tin roof.

There was an article I'd read recently about an artist famous for his vibrant colours who had become colour blind after a car accident and later confessed that he no longer even missed colour. Couldn't remember what he'd lost.

***

Doug and I walked down to the jetty in late-afternoon light, dark clouds gathering on the horizon. He wanted to catch squid for bait for the next blue-sky boating day. But I suspected it had more to do with his big heart. He wanted to ensure we did something together, even if it was a far cry from taking me out in his boat. He was prepared to regress to childhood and fish from a boring jetty. He was the iron man, with a soft heart.

He had a squid jag and a couple of spuds in a plastic bucket and I had a bottle of red wine and two glasses in a shoulder bag, and a plastic bag with cockles, handlines, and a fishing knife.

We were the only fools out and about. The beach and jetty were utterly deserted. The sky was threatening rain and although the wind was gusting around there was an uncanny feeling of being becalmed.

'We might catch a couple of crabs if nothing else,' I yelled to him as we cast out into different spots. I was convinced he'd gone mad. He was out at the very end of the jetty casting his squid jag into the jaws of the wind, Captain Ahab on his quest for Moby Dick.

He turned and yelled back: 'I've caught enough squid here at times to last me months.'

The moment my line hit bottom I knew we'd draw a blank. On the surface it looked perfect conditions for tommy ruff, but a strong current on the bottom was dragging the line around, snagging the hooks in weed. I wouldn't have felt a bite if I'd got one. I tried adding another sinker with no effect. An optimistic gull banked in the wind and hovered above the jetty, then swooped over the swell and landed on the beach. Lights from mansions above grey sandhills suggested sensible folk were cradling brandy balloons in front of roaring fires.

***

I spent Christmas night holed up in my room listening to an interview with Dad, recorded just before he died. It was comforting to once again hear the sound of the old man's frail voice, the whistling sibilance, and cracked high-pitched wheeze. Even the struggle for breath increased the illusion he was still alive. At one stage my brother came in and rummaged around in a chest of drawers, trying to interest me in sporting memorabilia that he shot out onto the bed behind me. But I was far more engrossed in my father's response to a question about what sort of games he'd played as a kid...

We used to make a toodlembuck out of a cotton reel and a piece of cardboard in the form of a circle divided up into sections. Some of the sections were wide, others narrow. And in the sections we'd write the names of famous race horses, like Carbine, Sassanoff, King & Goader, Night Marsh, and we'd put prices against them and spin the toodlembuck and there'd be a good chance of it coming against a wide space and that might be three to one. Whereas if it was on a narrow space where Carbine was, it'd be ten to one. And then we'd gamble from cigarette cards and if you won you might get three War Incident cards; the cigarette cards in those days when the war was on, showed war incidents – a series of cards in a cigarette pack...

I was listening with the spirit of a child who believes in alchemy, who believes that a real person is inside the radio, in this case the cassette player. Maybe magic was possible on a Christmas night. The excitation of magnetic particles on audiotape would conjure up his spirit, if not the man himself. In his last years, Dad reminded me of Marlon Brando in *The Godfather* in his last scene; in the orchard, going after his grandchild with the spraycan, scaring him with the same orange-peel teeth Dad wore to scare us. During one of our last family arguments, he'd wheezed out in his Don Corleone voice 'love one another'.

I began to sense the void again as my old man's answers trailed off. His voice faltered. Then Silence. Papers rustled and my nephew managed to crank-start the interview with a question about Dad's apprenticeship years.

Meanwhile Doug was still rummaging around in the bloody chest of drawers, as Dad was telling us about the joy of learning how to draw tools, then finding out that he was 'a natural' when it came to making the tools on fitting-and-turning machines. In response to a question about problems he had come across, you could almost hear the confidence coming back when he virtually dismissed the question out of hand. There was a *joy* in overcoming problems, don't you see?

I thought all this would appeal to the self-taught carpentry side of my brother; he had mastered the lathe and the thicknesser out in the shed, but he wouldn't sit beside me and just listen. He finally gave up on the memorabilia and wished me sweet dreams from the door.

As he was halfway out I said, 'Guess what Dad's last words were to me?'

'Make every post a winner?'

'No. Keep trying.'

While rewinding the tape to listen to his voice again, I recalled the unusual phone call I'd received from my surgeon's secretary just before coming here.

'We don't normally do this,' she'd said. 'But the doctor was wondering if you'd talk to one of our clients. He's not coping with his recent diagnosis. He's very upset.'

So I'd rung Glenn. He was fifty. He'd only been with the new girlfriend for six months. His main question was whether to take her on their planned trip to Hawaii over Christmas, or have the operation first. He told me his PSA was 15. Which was half what mine had been but well above my brother's. I advised him to have the holiday first. I told him the most important thing was to make love, without adding 'while you still can'.

Then I suddenly realised that I was spending Christmas night alone, obsessively listening to my father's voice – a man who'd managed to avoid doctors all his blessed life!

I went to bed and fiddled around in the dark, flicking at my flaccid member. Thinking of my young sister's psychic advice about 'imaging' a miracle, I kept on whipping my useless thing until I finally achieved a frog leg's spasm and the new 'post-coital' dull pain, with no wetness to confirm the event. The surgeon had never once brought up the psychological affect of suddenly experiencing only dry orgasms, which I imagined would seem an oxymoron to most men. He had only mentioned the ability to have an orgasm without an erection. This is the way the world ends, this is the way the world ends, not with a bang but a whimper.

I went to sleep thinking about Anna. Wanting to speak of many things. I would ratchet up my courage in Sydney and face what needed to be done. I would live without regret. I would live life passionately against the odds.

As I was going to sleep I managed a grin at the thought of Doug casting his squid jag into the wind. And then for some reason thought of the sixties television show *Laugh-In* and its corny refrain, *the fickle finger of fate.*

Next morning I rang JB to arrange an early ride back with him, then rebooked the flight to Sydney. I felt bad about abandoning Doug but I couldn't stand being away from Anna a minute longer. While driving to

Adelaide my oldest brother popped the question. My sister-in-law was driving their second car, so he seized the opportunity of having me to himself to ask the difference between our brother's PSA and mine.

I read between the lines. The question really meant that the word had spread. I wasn't handling it as well as my brother apparently had.

'*His* reading was just outside the safe zone, *mine* was through the roof.'

My pat reply didn't really hit the spot as far as I was concerned but it seemed to do the job.

'Ah,' he said, and sped up.

His wife was at a petrol station in Port Wakefield. I was about to follow JB into the toilet when she popped out of the café and gave me a long hug under the awnings. She was the only member of family who'd seen me in Sydney just before the operation. She'd flown up for a booked event with a girlfriend because my brother was unable to fly due to the bowel cancer. We had managed to avoid the topic of my operation until Anna left the kitchen. Then I took the bull by the horns and said, 'I think I might as well *leave* her after the operation.'

'What? And become a hermit? That doesn't sound like you, Pierre.'

PART TWO

11

Anna came into view as I was riding the escalator to baggage collection. We hugged as if nothing out of the ordinary had happened in 2008. On New Year's Eve anything is possible.

The drive home from the airport was anti-climactic after the introspection during my pilgrimage. I heard about how she'd caught up on sleep at her sister's over Christmas and played marathon Scrabble games.

We were soon driving over Anzac Bridge, a salmon-pink sky on the western horizon. A whiff of the fish markets. The new sculpture 'The Soldier' flashed past, and I was back on the peninsula known for its staunch Labor tradition and 'Balmain boys don't cry' in the face of defeat, from the rugby league ovals to the polling booths.

We went out onto the lower deck, the lunatic asylum tower alight above the tree line like a beacon of hope. The possums had almost stripped the wild avocado tree. I put a banana out for them anyway. The look of trust in the mum's brown doe-eyes whenever she materialised out of the darkness at the first hint of candlelight, made me feel blessed that Mother Nature could be alive and well in the land of whipper snippers, chainsaws and angle grinders. 'Our' possum would let Anna touch her as she sat on her haunches, hypnotically nibbling a banana, huge bushy tail draped over the balustrade.

I picked up Puss and gave her a cuddle. She'd been playing hard to get ever since I'd walked in the door. I put Bach on and a chorus of frogs joined in. We toasted in the New Year with a bottle of bubbly. 'Here's to not going gently into that good night,' I said.

'Here's to us,' Anna responded.

I felt happier than I had in months, almost as if I was back in my skin. We looked at a family photo album I'd unearthed at Doug's. Anna honed in on a sepia print of me as a baby, with snowy white hair. I would've been about a year old. Then the eight-year-old version: knock-kneed, wearing hand-me-down shorts, arms laced through gaps in the wrought-iron front gate.

'I can see why your mum loved you to bits,' Anna said. 'She told me that you know.'

I told her that Mum had loved *her* the moment she laid eyes on her. Anna asked how I knew, and I told her I just did.

'Doug loves you too,' she said, 'even if he sometimes seems like a rusty old spring.'

'I know. I felt I was abandoning him by going back earlier than planned. I was just so sick of all that unspoken stoicism. He wanted to see the old me back. As if nothing has changed.'

'Why didn't you talk to him?'

'It was up to him.'

'What would you have said if he had?'

'I don't know. "All the signs are good." Leave it at that.'

Anna's phone rang. She let it ring for a while before going to get it. 'That'll be my sister. I'll try and make it brief.'

'Put on the short dress and the knickers I bought for you,' I said. She glanced over her shoulder and mimed an exaggerated kiss with her beautiful lips.

I sipped champagne and thought about her. She had never been a short-dress type of girl. Although a female friend at one of our parties had once said – as Anna was perched on the kitchen bench, legs dangling – 'I'd never thought of you as having such shapely legs, Anna.'

The sheer black stockings may have had a bit to do with it that night but it was more her uncharacteristic flaunting of female freedom. Wearing a dress and that sensual contact of air on skin is a freedom denied men. I knew penetrative sex was out of the question but I was looking forward to getting on with my rehabilitation after seeing the surgeon.

When she walked onto the deck in candlelight, in the diaphanous dress, I knew why I'd bought the outfit for her. It was straight out of a Bettina Arndt script but I'd take it.

'I'm wearing the pants you bought me,' she said. She bent down and kissed me. I lifted the dress and touched the dark curve of satin. I stood and we kissed, the decadent taste of fresh cigarette on her breath. Her body felt ethereal, liberated by physical contact from last year's bad karma. Her mound of Venus had a mnemonic effect, an ancient flicker of the flame. I'd seen that light in her eyes before, when we first made love, as she'd arched up under me.

'You seem like a new man,' she said. We stood united, kissing, the New Year's fireworks kicking in.

***

Next morning two wine glasses were still on the deck surrounded by the aluminium cups with their burnt-out tea lights. The photo album was still open at the baby shot, protected by half a century of rice paper. I tidied up the table and swept the deck and sat down. Last night I'd seemed like 'a new man' according to Anna.

There was little to our tiny backyard but the avocado tree. Originally a potted gift from one of Anna's female friends, it had grown into a beautiful wild thing that softened the glare from a neighbour's second storey addition.

I sat down where we'd celebrated the New Year on my return, but I hadn't really come back. I was not the same person who sat here last year blissfully unaware of what was just around the corner. Last night we'd made do with a kiss and a cuddle in bed despite the sexual summer night's dreaming on this balcony, a balcony that now seemed sexless and bland.

For the rest of the morning I worked my way through the accumulated emails. January would be unusually busy, starting tomorrow afternoon. A couple from New Zealand, celebrating their engagement, had booked a portrait shoot in the Chinese Gardens back in October, and relieved to be free of the catheter and the urine bag strapped to my thigh, I had automatically made the booking.

Anna drove me to the location. I felt like I was going mad. Two days back and we weren't talking. The morning peace and quiet on the deck had been brutally shattered by the neighbours' roller door. Rolling over everything like a Russian tank's surprise invasion of Prague. I felt under siege. Not even Anna had understood. We got along well enough with our neighbours – apart from the felling of a tree or the cutting back of the bougainvillea. So I couldn't explain my erratic behaviour in words. I'd slammed the door and rushed back inside, throwing the newspaper to the floor. Nothing rational. A roller door is just a roller door. It was the sound that did it...

I thought back to an old English teacher whose fragile mental state had been caused by shellshock from the Second World War. Whenever workmen carried out school maintenance and started banging their hammers, he would throw his poetry book on the desk and wince as he covered his ears.

After crossing Anzac Bridge we idled at the lights and then drove towards the Chinese Garden of Friendship. I held onto the sweet sound of the ABC Classic FM announcer's voice, the woman with the endearing slight lisp. A while ago I'd discovered she was a viola player and had short auburn hair and was a lesbian to boot. The latter only increased her appeal because I had assumed her life was the formulaic breeze of the bourgeois blonde. But I'd fallen in love with the sound of her voice.

She dropped me off outside the gardens on an unfamiliar stretch of road as alienating as Jeffrey Smart's painting, *Cahill Expressway.* I was that figure, plunked down in an artificial-looking cityscape. Scaled down after bleak surgical excavations.

I found the steps leading up to a café that fitted the description of the rendezvous point. When they walked up, an old part of me unconsciously kicked in and I struggled to my feet and shook their hands. I had the presence of mind to suggest a table where we could discuss poses. Snap-happy Japanese were swarming around like ants, draping themselves over bridges, craning to get shots of mini-rapids and generally posing everywhere. So I led my young clients off the beaten track into a grove of trees, to avoid a nervous breakdown as much as the Japanese, and where people wouldn't be able to insinuate themselves into the background. I gradually warmed to them, and composed a series of intimate portraits by rapids. I arranged to email a short list of low-resolution images they could choose from as they left to catch a cab to Manly and felt a load lift from my shoulders. I'd survived the first day back in the work-a-day world post-operation.

12

The sound of the door shutting as Anna left for work woke me. I went to the toilet and then tried to get back to sleep but voices from my 'holiday' kept going round and round in my head.

I went downstairs and brewed coffee. It was too early to console myself with the Test on television between Australia and South Africa, but out on the deck I felt refreshed after a precious one-and-a-half hour's sleep-in. A white butterfly flitted through the broad green leaves of the avocado tree, and then settled on the twig of a dead pot plant on the deck. My gaze drifted to a stain in the woodwork where I'd left my DNA imprint a year ago; a balmy summer's night when, on a lonely impulse, I'd masturbated out here when Anna was away overseas.

The pool is just a short drive away. The ritualistic lap-swimming helped keep my demons at bay. Looking down from the bleachers to the lanes, the place, still unpretentious fifties architecture, had charm. The glinting water, lap swimmers, readers and topless sunworshippers over on the grass. Glimpses of sandstone buildings across the water in the old lunatic asylum grounds, and yachts moored in the cove.

I changed into my bathers, using a towel around my waist, and went down the stone steps shaded by the majestic Moreton Bay fig. It was a good time of day.

No lanes off-limits for swimming classes, just modern youth bomb-diving from the edge of the bubble and shriek lane to impress the girls.

I exercised on Spartan wooden slats by the wading pool and then did my regime of anal clenches on the side of the pool before dropping like a stone. After twenty laps, I hauled myself out and sat at the edge of the pool, seawater sloshing around in the gutters, smudges of white cloud in the sky – 'above us only sky' as Lennon sang – and the occasional car clanking across Iron Cove Bridge.

There was not another soul in the blissful cement silence of the men's cramped change room. This is where I used to come ten years ago, after Anna's miscarriage, to find solace as much as to swim. A screaming kid broke the silence. His father's pathetic attempt to quieten him had no effect at all. The awful high-pitched sound kept going, on and on, echoing around and around, cancelling any spiritual gain from my swim.

Sitting outside Café Lazio in downtown Rozelle rekindled the feeling of strength from the solitude of swimming. The coffee acted as a catalyst to keep my armour in place, to keep thoughts of the future at bay. Wanting my family to ask how I was but, paradoxically, not to ask. Finally understanding what Hemingway had meant when he said: 'There are many ways families can be dangerous.'

***

I got a call from my surgeon's secretary to put off the appointment for the first post-operative PSA test results. A reprieve. I tried staying busy as one brother had advised, but couldn't quite manage to 'move on' as another implied I should. I was only going into the Outside World for real-estate photography jobs. I tried not to think about the worst-case scenario: cancer cells spreading in spite of the radical measures taken; then radiation, the 'second bite at the cherry'. Despite the surgeon's god-like status in my eyes, I knew even he could have got it wrong.

Driving around the harbour, I almost forgot what had happened, but whenever I was hurrying against the dying of the light or negotiating lifts with swipe cards in underground car parks, the void would return. The first bill from pathology didn't help. It reminded me that these blood tests would be hanging round my neck for a while, possibly for the rest of my life.

Glenn rang to thank me for advising him to go on the Hawaiian holiday before having the operation. He had opted to have robotics despite my recommending our traditional surgeon. I wasn't against robotics, as such. He was on sick leave and he'd been surfing the Internet about post-prostatectomy issues. He promised to email me his findings. 'You've helped me so I'll help you,' he said. 'From now on we're travelling the same road together.'

I was touched. I was his new brother-at-arms. He wished me luck for my PSA result and we made a date to have coffee and finally meet face-to-face. The closer the appointment with my surgeon loomed, the more my fear of death took precedence over my fear of a sexless future.

One day, while looking out over the park from the upstairs window, the backwash of traffic along Victoria Road a comforting, almost oceanic presence, I remembered a recent dream. I was on an old-fashioned hospital bed, floating above the ocean, the water far below like crenulated velvet. Then I was back on the edge of my father's sick bed, with his last words to me. *Keep trying.*

13

Anna had taken Friday afternoon off to accompany me to the surgeon's rooms for the first post-operation PSA test result, even though I'd told her she shouldn't feel obliged to come. But I was glad to have her by my side, in case of bad news. I'd read somewhere that the operation *itself* could cause long dormant cancer cells to be released into your bloodstream. I'd also read an article in favour of 'watchful waiting'. When our surgeon told me after the operation, 'I think you've had this a very long time' I chose to think he meant it was just as well we got it when we did.

When the appointment had been made in the New Year to see my surgeon, it had felt a long way off in a 'safe' future. At least this time we could park in a suburban street rather than in the hospital's all-day car park, as we had to on D Day. We held hands and walked under lime-green trees in morning sun, up the steps into the building. We stopped holding hands outside the victims' lift. It automatically descended to the basement, which felt a bad sign, before going back to where we'd started.

We got out at infamous Level Three and walked past the honey-coloured doors bearing the names of medical specialists. One was ajar enough for a glimpse of white coats huddled around screens in a room lit by soulless fluorescent lighting. A snatch of laughter followed us along the interminable corridor before we arrived at the only door that mattered.

I opened the door and ushered Anna in first. An old man was by the counter paying the secretary. I sat down and looked at the paintings on the wall, the same serene blue-and-white scenes from Greek Islands we saw nine months ago when we first came. I had no doubt the paintings were chosen to keep us thinking positively about the future, all those holidays in Europe to look forward to, when the hurly-burly was done, the battle lost and won.

The secretary seemed to avoid looking at me, even after the old man had left. I feared the worst. She was cradling her phone, only her head visible behind the high reception counter. She looked objective, as if we were no more than customers at a checkout in a supermarket about to be barcode-scanned, tallied up, and checked for Fly Buys. It was difficult to associate her with the woman who'd phoned, apologetic about asking me to talk to Glenn.

A good-looking Italian woman entered with her son. He would've been no more than nineteen, wearing crisp blue jeans with iconoclastic creases ironed into them by his mother. They sat in a corner by a vase of orange tiger lilies, a quilt of pollen around the base. My heart went out to her handsome son, doomed at such a young age to share a room with middle-aged men. He clutched a sheaf of scans to his chest like a shield. She wore a brave blank mask and stared straight ahead. Poor woman. Poor boy.

I stared at the floor until the wood blurred into hypnotic patterns. Then the door opened and I heard my name as the bottom of a white coat swept across to reception. Anna was already halfway to the door when I stood up and followed.

We sat down on the other side of an uncluttered desk. No preliminaries this time. He looked at some papers, then up at me and smiled.

'Your PSA is fine: 0.006. Virtually undetectable.'

I punched the air and hissed out *yes.*

I was completely overcome with relief. From 35 to 0.006! It seemed to vindicate the decision. Anna had tears in her eyes as I reached out to her. We held hands. Tightly. It had been the first good news in ten months. Nothing else mattered as far as I was concerned. I would not have to undergo radiation, at least not yet.

The rest of the consultation passed in a pleasant blur. I answered questions as if applying for a job. No, I wasn't experiencing any difficulty urinating *but* I *was* using a wad of toilet paper in my underpants on photography gigs, probably psychological? Our surgeon agreed. I should stop doing that.

'How are the erections?' he asked.

I'd been waiting for that one. The ridiculous TV ad about men's health, set in a doctor's consultation room, the white elephant in the background looking over the patient's shoulder, invisible only to the patient.

'They're non-existent,' I said, straight up. 'I experience a lengthening and a swelling if I whip it around masturbating. But as you said, at least it's possible to have an orgasm without an erection.'

I knew Anna wouldn't mind the men's business. It would be water off a duck's back to her compared to living with my depression. Our surgeon was not like some specialists I'd read about on Glenn's internet blogs, who take their patients' grief personally. An uncaring version of the Hippocratic oath: 'Well, what do you expect *me* to do about it? I got rid of your cancer, what more do you want?'

Fortunately we'd chosen a humanitarian.

'I've found that nearly all my patients who have had a radical prostatectomy don't even think about sex for the first six months. They're usually too busy recovering from the operation itself and handling incontinence issues,' he explained. 'You've done really well on that front. But the sooner you start injecting the better.'

He wrote a referral for a doctor in another hospital where I could get the penile injection lessons for free. He said it was a necessary part of my sexual rehab.

The injections would apparently promote blood flow in the spongy tissue of the penis where the magical stiffening happens – or happened in my case. It would help to stop the scar tissue that would lead to permanent erectile dysfunction – *impotence.*

He had already told us that Viagra was completely ineffective after a radical prostatectomy but he wrote out a prescription for the new sex pills anyway. 'You just never know,' he said.

Until then I'd associated penile injections with *other* surgeons, having always believed mine would spare enough nerves for Mother Nature to eventually come back. I hadn't realised that injecting had a role in rehabilitation. I was hearing about cold steel in my dick to help the promotion of oxygen and 'using it or losing it'. I resisted.

Injecting seemed like an admission of defeat. I clung to the possibility that my old football fitness and middle-aged swimming and tennis would be my ultimate healer. And time would eventually vindicate my decision to put faith in *this s* urgeon and no other.

We shook hands before leaving. I think Anna wanted to kiss him. The secretary wrote out the referral for the next PSA test in three months. I didn't bother mentioning Glenn to her. It might've sounded like I wanted a medal.

We walked quickly along the corridor holding hands. The sun streamed in through the windows as we waited for the lift. Even the hospital grounds on the opposite side of the road, where the deed had been done, looked quite beautiful. From the third floor the world suddenly seemed a different place. I could just make out the flat roof decorated in white pebbles that I'd stared at from my hospital bed for three days. Woodstock, the hippie rock event of the century, also took three days to change the world. In a strange way it felt as if it had never happened, a bad dream. I would never have allowed myself to be butchered like that surely? One day as strong as a bull, three days later a cripple. Why would any 'free spirit' *ever* decide to do that? The lift was empty. We kissed. Then walked into the street talking of going to a pub to celebrate.

'I can't believe it. I'd been expecting bad news,' I said, slowing down to keep holding her hand.

'I knew it was good news the moment he called your name. He smiled at us so warmly.'

'Did he? I couldn't bear to look. I was steeling myself, with the readings I had, to be told I'd need radiation.'

'*Had,* my love, had. But now, 'virtually undetectable'. I always knew we'd chosen the right man.'

We drove to the Riverview Hotel, the pub Dawn Fraser had famously owned. The other local contender, The Bald Rock, was probably unconsciously ruled out due to the negative associations from the night we went there to chew the fat after the second PSA result, and then to drown our sorrows after the killer biopsy result when I walked out of the beer garden into the dusk. The wine and brandy had stopped working and I stood in the middle of the road and told Anna and the parked cars, and the street, and the sky, and the universe, and anyone else interested that I intended doing *fucking nothing!* Later that night Anna reiterated her support for whatever decision I made. Might it have been better to party on? We'd never know.

The Riverview was close to the courts where we played tennis each week. It was the only social outlet that allowed me to push *it* into the background for an hour. I enjoyed teaching Anna nearly as much as I did playing. It somehow united us in a way that nothing else had over the previous year. The pub was uncrowded for a Friday afternoon. It had moved with the times. A new curved bar had replaced the old box-like style and there was a more upmarket, less bohemian clientele to match the new design. We took two fluted glasses of champagne to the lounge room and sat in a brand new pink leather couch.

Anna proposed a toast. 'I knew Paul was the one from the very first meeting. Quite apart from his one hundred per cent statistics for preventing incontinence,' she said.

The place began to fill with post-work patrons, so we went upstairs to a small courtyard with a view over Balmain rooftops. I got another round of champagne and Anna proposed a second toast.

'Here's to our angel. For not only being a great surgeon, but a darling man!'

She raised her glass.

It must've been the sudden realisation that we were toasting an ordinary man with an ordinary name – a man who had wiped out my manhood. Was everything hunky-dory now? Were we back to 'normal' now because I wasn't pissing myself in public?

I suddenly felt nothing but anger.

Not one person had opposed my caving in to the operation. Not one person even planted a seed of doubt. I didn't respond to the toast. I held the glass tightly on the table by its fucking fragile stem.

'I wish I'd never met him,' I said. 'I don't know how you could've gone along with such a barbaric act. I might as well go and live in a tent on the Nullarbor.'

We drove home in silence.

I'd been made aware of the surgeon's priorities. He'd made them crystal clear: cancer, incontinence, nerve sparing. In that practical, descending, hierarchal, order.

I don't know why I spoilt the day. I knew I was doing exactly what the conservative brochures I'd be given in hospital had warned me about. Taking it out on those nearest and dearest to you. It was the brutality I needed to out. Of course I wish I'd never met him! But paradoxically he was everything Anna had gushed about.

When we got home, I went straight upstairs and sat at my lookout post, staring at the old lunatic asylum tower, punishing Anna for her complicity with the butchers. But when the front door slammed I knew she'd go to her mum's place a suburb away. Maybe she'd stay the night this time, though she'd never resorted to that before.

As the hours went by I sat upstairs staring at the dimly lit mad person's tower on the other side of the park, wondering if I'd finally succeeded in driving her away. But I kept reminding myself that I had *not* been incontinent *or* impotent *before* the diagnosis. I'd been 'cured' of something that wasn't wrong with me in the first place. Other than the relatively minor matter of a slow stream, never a serious quality-of-life issue, apart from interrupted sleep.

I began to think of the row as the precursor to breaking up.

Over the past ten years we'd rarely argued, apart from one or two silly political disagreements. She had her mother's sense of Irish injustice, of siding with the underdog, but didn't fly off the handle as easily as her mum. When she did, Anna was capable of slaying dragons.

I heard her come in through the front door downstairs without her usual 'yoo-hoo!' greeting. I hurried down to apologise. She was sitting with her head over a newspaper at the kitchen table and didn't look up as I came down the hallway. I sat and put my hand over hers, as I had with my dad the last time I saw him alive.

'I'm really sorry. You're the last person I want to hurt. I think when I said "I wish I'd never met him" it was a kind of release valve. Does that make any sense?'

She squeezed my hand and looked at me with those beautiful, otherworldly humane blue eyes. 'Of course it makes sense. I just needed to be with the wise old owl for a while. I didn't say anything to her.'

She had forgiven me.

I hadn't realised how much stress she'd been under because of me. Not to mention looking after an ageing mum who was virtually bedridden and blind. Anna was the personification of the opposite of cruel to be kind. Such a merciful woman to have in my life, whatever was left of this 'beautiful life', as the bloke in the hospital bed next to mine called it. When I went over to shake his hand and say goodbye he said: 'And don't worry about that *other* thing. There's much more to this beautiful life than sex.'

I realised he must've overheard me crying to the nurse that first night, and the coded conversation with the surgeon two days later. Though when he said it, my instinctive reaction was, *what* is more beautiful than sex – sunsets, paintings by Vermeer? As aesthetically inspiring as the contemplation of beauty may be, it does not have the same affect on my life force as sex. Only dead people don't have sex.

I knew there was something wrong with me, which went deeper than a surgeon's blade. Very few women would have stuck around. A few weeks after my return from the pilgrimage, Anna again suggested that I 'see someone'. She knew a lot about mental health because she had studied it. We were both interested in Jung. But going to see a therapist still seemed to me to be grasping at straws when, before all this, I had been happy and self-confident.

'I'm really worried about us, Pete,' she said. 'I know you're hurting, but we need to be kind to each other.' (When she'd walked out, I'd yelled down the stairs: 'Yeah that's right, run away to your mother's place. You spend more time there than you do on my fucking rehabilitation!')

Why not some joy for her now? Why had I not danced, glass of champagne in hand, at the Riverview? Perhaps because I was still wondering where this modern medical management was leading. To the subliminal S-bend in the toilet of the mind I suspected. Keep the stink submerged. Cover it with linguistic disinfectants: move on, get over it, the cancer journey, have a nice day, no problem. I had begun to blame her for her passive role in it. I had threatened to leave her and go back to the desert because I felt I had been made into a mathematical figure, a zero point zero zero six.

The next day I sent a thank you card to our surgeon, as Anna had suggested. Then I bought my first packet of Viagra with his prescription – *you just never know.* I chose a chemist warehouse (as opposed to whorehouse) a couple of suburbs away. Not because the four-pill packet would cost seventy-eight dollars instead of eighty-five dollars, but because the local chemist knew me, and I wanted to avoid the personal stigma. I followed a sign to a counter down the far end of a supermarket-sized pharmacology section and handed the script to a young man in the ubiquitous white coat. Five minutes later I took a metal tray containing a tiny box to the checkout. Something I would eventually accept as normal, along with the expense, as part and parcel of a man's ineluctable, non-tax-deductible treatment.

***

It was the last day of Anna's holidays. We had planned to get up early and go to a surf beach, something we hadn't done since waiting for the biopsy results at Bundeena on my fifty-ninth birthday. I could hear her up and about downstairs and decided to pop a Viagra and try sex, maybe go to the beach on a miraculous high. Knowing the pill took an hour to work I went to the bathroom and, without letting Anna know, took a tablet and crept back to bed.

I woke with the most promising swelling I'd had since the operation and flicked at the shape inside my jocks and then whipped it against my belly. The swelling increased, suggesting that even though there was no hardness, *some* nerves must've been spared.

Anna was reading a novel at the kitchen table when I appeared in my new Calvin Klein's. Her eyes went straight there and she smiled.

'I took Viagra an hour ago. Do you want to have sex and then go the beach?'

She reached out and I walked up.

'Mm, yes I'd like that,' she said. There was a sexual burr to her voice. I felt her feathered touch.

'Give me a few minutes and then come up. Wear the panties I bought for you in Adelaide.'

'I'd love to wear them,' she said. I knew she was indulging me. But the mnemonic word conjured up sex. Call it a pornographic catalyst for the chthonic, or what fanatical feminists term the *infantalisation* of women, but even conjuring the idea of their smaller – compared with men's – underwear, had arousal potential. There would be time for ideological re-education camps after I'd recovered my manhood. Right now it was whatever it took.

The warnings about possible side effects inside the Viagra packet were long enough to extend to the floor. But for me there was just a fuzzy halo around the edge of the television screen and a slight facial flush. I went to the computer and adjusted the screen so that I could see the bulge and the almost hallucinogenic blue fuzziness. I stood there self-consciously anticipating Anna coming in, but managed to produce a good length rather than good *line and* length – as they say of a fast bowler in cricketing parlance.

The door opened and Anna came in wearing a black top and the pornographic pure white panties. We embraced and I pressed myself into her. I could tell she didn't know what to do after feeling my uncertainty. She probably wanted me to fuck her over the bed like a chemical stud, but instead asked what I wanted her to do. I told her to get onto the bed so I could look at her. She lay down and started to make tiny circles over the silken fabric. I felt a slight response. She squatted in front of me but I stopped her from trying fellatio. I knew I was still too soft. I asked her to get into doggie position and squatted behind her and 'imaged' a miracle. I whipped my hose against her sacrificial rump with her knickers pulled back and touched her between her smooth legs as her hand snaked back to feel me.

I tried to focus on the earlier world of fantasy, even though I knew I should verbalise it. But I wasn't ready to do that despite the Lord having famously said: 'First there was the Word then the Word was made Flesh.'

I was human, all too human. I had no idea without the old hardness. So I asked her to be rougher. 'Don't change a thing,' I said, spelling out the simple male desire for repetition. You just never know.

14

Coogee Beach was a piece of theatre. A white apron before a blue-green ocean, waves glinting in the sun under a child's blue sky.

We chose a spot in the shade by the sea wall. I felt what could only be described as the first feeling of communal happiness to come over me in a long time. I watched her strip down to her one-piece black bathing suit. I lay there on my towel next to my woman and read the paper, but my eyes kept drifting to Anna's pear-shaped arse. Which only a few hours ago had been in my face, squatting on our bed after months of nothingness. Even though, in the end, I hadn't been able to enter her. At a high school swimming carnival she'd once beaten a girl who would go on to win Olympic gold. I felt happy to be on the beach with my dark star. A taste of sexual intimacy was all it had taken, even just the attempt.

Thirty metres down the beach a group of young Japanese were having trouble erecting an umbrella in the strong breeze that had sprung up. I watched this beautiful couple. She was in a skimpy black bikini. He was wearing below-the-knee board shorts. In enormous sunglasses, they had metamorphosed into insect heads. The others were doing a bizarre combination of beach stomp and slow motion Noh play. Lying down on the sand one minute, springing up and swooping across the beach like a seagull the next. Then they all came together to form a daisy chain and walked to the water holding hands. They stood at the edge, statues silhouetted in blue light.

I thought about our sex a few hours ago, after which I'd happily gone to Balmain to do the shopping. I'd browsed in a bookshop feeling the strange new Viagra optimism, an aberrant purple-blue rim around my sunglasses as I floated across the road to the Unity Hall Hotel. The entire world had a pleasant purple haze. My slightly blocked nose did not feel unpleasant, but only reminded me of our sex.

I urinated with a strong stream and took a glass of water to a dimly lit ledge and watched an old man at a table by the window, nursing a schooner of beer. Then I took the sliding door exit into Beattie Street and walked to the car feeling as if nothing much was wrong with the world.

The Viagra sex had ultimately been a failure but it had brought us to this pure white sand, to this beach. We approached the ocean holding hands. The water was achingly cold and the waves were breaking too close to shore to body surf. We drifted blissfully around in the water out the back.

After collecting our things we went in search of better waves. I followed Anna's directions down obscure streets, hugging the cliffs to stay close to the oceanic feeling. Like following our noses in France, trusting pastoral fairies would direct us to an idyllic picnic spot where we'd put our world to rights over local wine, cheeses, tomatoes, and olives. But we eventually got sick of driving into dead ends and finished up at Bronte.

It was packed.

We settled for a one-hour meter on the serpentine split-level road at the northern end and walked down the esplanade glimpsing emerald-green waves through the forest of trees leading down to Dylan's circus sands.

The whole beach rolled into view.

I wanted to get there as quickly as possible, for Anna to run free with me down the grassy slope. But not having my goat legs or mind, she took the long way via the steps while I slid down the slope. I reached the lawn and watched her descend in the white dress I'd bought for her in Adelaide. Until today, she'd only ever worn it on New Year's Eve, along with the knickers that would be in the laundry after this morning's session. The breeze blew her dress up and exposed a flash of peaches and cream thigh as she came down the path with her red and orange bohemian bag. I sensed that *the thing* might become, if not a good thing, then at least something that might ironically bring us closer sexually.

She took my arm and we floated down the path to the caves under the cliffs. We found a spot on the yellow sand set back from the madding crowd and laid the towels out there. Then we walked down to the water holding hands and got lost in the surf midst the jumble of bodies and white water and undertow. She was having a ball. Once, during a lull, we hugged. But the water was too cold for anything mystical to occur below the belt. There would be no reverse psychology overcoming the male shrinkage factor; no manifestation of a magical underwater erection, as might've happened in former times – and which I still hoped might happen again if I didn't think about it.

After that first water-friendly hug, I let go of the idea. It was expecting too much too soon. I felt as if the Viagra may be having a perverse anti-shrinkage effect. But it was so cold I couldn't stay in long enough to investigate any further and Anna had already been hero enough for one day.

While towelling off on the beach my gaze latched onto a young topless woman lying on her stomach reading, her sculpted vertebrae and the taut brown skin forming a gentle slope from her shoulders all the way down to her generous buttocks, to the abstruse line of the vulva in the shadow of her clinging bikini bottoms.

I remembered the parking meter and looked out to sea and located my seal pup still amongst the waves. I forced my way out to her through a strong undertow, bordering on rip. The tide had turned and the waves were starting to dump. Something had also shut down in me in spite of all her watery glory.

I ran back up the slope and then walked at a pace that reminded me of my sister walking to the beach with me, leaving me for dust. Sure enough the zombies had struck. The parking ticket was huge. The fascist Waverley Council was alive and well. Anna arrived and saw the ticket I'd left there under the wiper.

'We should've gone earlier,' I said. 'It was freezing on the beach.'

'Let's not allow a parking fine to spoil the day. I'll pay,' she said.

'No you won't. I will. Let's just go home.'

The black cloud had descended and there was nothing I could do. I had insisted on paying for doctors' bills, blood tests, and sex pills, anything to do with my bad karma. Perhaps it would be nice to pay for something that was bad in a normal way, just for once – but it had drained the colour from the day in an instant.

A board outside a pub announced 'Beer battered fish and chips'. I swung into a park. We ordered and took glasses of wine into the beer garden. A beautiful young woman walked past in a white bikini and tank top, and an African man strode on the lower path, a coffee-coloured baby in his arms. The couple rammed home the emptiness, the finite nature of the annihilation. A few hours on a beach towel and fooling in the surf had all been washed away as easily as a kid's sandcastle. The sex this morning really only stirred up what was missing. The couple and the baby confirmed it.

I imagined dating again, my secret sexuality fighting against my shrivelled-up world. We'd passed some sort of milestone this morning but it was the milestone of a small world. I recalled our passionate first months, visiting a friend of Anna's on the central coast. On the way home we went to the surf beach together. There were just dumpers that day. But I'd gone in anyway to impress Anna. Afterwards as we sat outside a café back from the beach, a flash of white underwear, a second of touching her under the table. Visiting a local jazz festival on the way home, and making love against a gum tree as golden trumpet notes floated across the village green.

***

On the way home Anna caught every red light. I could feel her stiff compliance as I willed her to beat them. Only after entering the sanctuary of our home and sliding down at the table could I begin to join the post-Coogee Beach dots.

Anna put a chicken in the oven and chopped vegetables. I drank a glass of red wine and watched her. Then finally plucked up the courage to speak.

'I'm really sorry,' I blurted out. She stopped chopping and came over and sat down.

'It was great at Coogee. But then something happened. I don't know quite what. I wanted to go home but you stayed in the water too long.'

'I wish you'd told me you'd had enough.'

'You were making the most of the last day of your holidays.'

'So that's why you got so stressed out on the way home? I thought it was the parking ticket.'

'That was the straw that broke the camel's back. Coogee was enough of being back in the world for one day. The rest just reminded me how unreal the world has become. I can't seem to shake the feeling that I made the wrong decision, that I should've stuck to my guns, stayed whole, and accepted death.'

'It's too late to think like that now. Remember how you said you didn't think you could handle always worrying about whether the cancer was spreading. That nagging feeling – remember? So you'll just have to tell me when that eggshell fragility of yours needs returning to its nest. I actually think you've been unhappy for a long time.'

'No, that's not it,' I protested. 'I haven't been unhappy for a long time. I've been up and down like anyone else. You're quite wrong there. This is something altogether new for fuck's sake. Can't you see? I'm pining for a desert where nobody knows me.'

'I know,' she said, maybe having had second thoughts about my irreversible decision herself, but not letting on.

At least with a vasectomy there was the chance of untying the knot. But the mind is not so easily unknotted. She was pointing out that I had a tendency to depression, trying to put it all *in perspective.*

'I love you so very much,' she said against the grain. 'We had a lovely day until then. We made love. The signs are all good, as you say. I feel closer to you when we get physically close.'

I felt a tear slide down a cheek, something in the memory about more to this beautiful life than sex. For me it had to do with honesty. For women it apparently had nothing to do with sex per se. She had grown up surrounded by literature and had read voraciously. After finishing an arts degree in archaeology she worked for seven years at Penguin Books and was offered training as an editor, but didn't wish to move to Melbourne. She had always been my go-to-person before I sent my short stories to competitions, or important photographic jobs to clients. She had a strong editorial ear for prose, and an unerring eye in the visual arts.

'I also need to tell you that I feel bad about how I used you in bed this morning,' I said to this intelligent woman, my faithful sexual partner of ten years as well as my unsung muse.

'Don't feel bad. I love being intimate with you.'

'I think I'll go and see a dick doctor about the injections. The Man said "use it or lose it".'

'I could get off on watching you inject. It could be quite a turn on.'

It had come from out of the blue. She sounded like the flower-power child she would've been had she been born a decade earlier. I topped up her glass and imagined her watching me inject, imagined injecting period. Knowing my editor was on the same unwritten page as me made all the difference, all the difference in the world.

15

I still woke to the disappointment of no erections in the morning and the gradual realisation that I might never wake with another hard-on ever again. Once it had been our main time for spontaneous sex. I'd had a dream. Anna had her suitcase packed and the old bloke in the hospital bed next to mine said there's much more to this beautiful life than sex. We were at a party. My guitar fell to the floor and the neck cracked and broke off from the body.

I eventually got up, made toast, and went back upstairs to gaze out at the tower. The fan cooled my naked back and I suddenly wanted to ring all the people I'd cut over the last six months. They'd sensed defeat in the tone of my voice over the phone, and had never rung back. Wishing the old confident persona back. Some might say the too-confident character based on my previous life as footy star, the mask that for all my attempts, I had never quite managed to lose.

An erstwhile schoolmate had recently self-published a novella with a minor character known as 'the legend' based on me. In a scene set in the late nineties when I had been living alone in Elizabeth Bay near Kings Cross, I was described as the sort of person who left his door unlocked in an ex-hotel converted into flats full of junkies. According to the writer, after my triumphs in my short but legendary Aussie Rules career, including 'winning a Grand Final off his own boot', he'd written that I'd thought of myself as so special as to be beyond the wrath of God, or words to that affect. I knew enough about fiction to realise that he was using hyperbole to boost the emotional tenor of his story. And I took being dubbed 'the legend' with a grain of salt as well. I'd gone out of my way back then, to avoid fans. A brother of mine would later suggest, I'd gone too far out of my way. I'd proved him right by disappearing into another orbit altogether after marrying too young and joining the hippies up north. Or maybe that had become my convenient alibi over the years.

I knew it was no fictional exaggeration to say Anna and I had become ships in the night since the failed Viagra attempt. I was finding it increasingly difficult to find the motivation to even get up, and go for a swim in the mornings, to start the long empty days on a positive note.

One day after Anna had gone to teach she left me a note on the kitchen table telling me to 'have a good one'. It was hot and steamy on the deck and the cicadas were buzzing like witchdoctors exorcising the air of evil spirits. I told myself to stop pushing her away. Stop giving her more reasons to split up than she already had. Why couldn't I just accept the loss of sex?

I went to the bathroom and grabbed the Viagra packet from the cabinet, tore out a pill, and drank it down with a glass of water. In the bedroom I drew the curtains, undressed and turned on the television. I folded the doona back and lay on the bed, watching mindlessly for half an hour.

The blue aura appeared around the screen and there was a definite swelling in my jocks. I wasn't expecting a miracle second time round, but you just never knew, as the surgeon said.

I squatted over the pillow and flicked at my swollen dick. My rubbery thing lengthened with every fantasy, and, with intense concentration and my stomach muscles flexed at the same time as relaxing my pelvic floor, I could get a swelling with a tenuous component of hardness. But within a few seconds of my member teasing me with the memory of its true shape I came half a second after the illusion of being a man once again.

I tried to go to sleep but kept thinking about my relationship with Anna. I wanted it to be biased towards sex. But this was going to be a long haul. I'd only been able to achieve a fraction of the hardness required for penetration. And I'd read all the literature on the various substitutes for traditional sex including soft-entry techniques with the woman on top – nothing new to someone from the sixties sexual revolution. Most men and women use fantasy in sex. But since that first platonic night on New Year's Eve when we'd finished up in bed with a kiss and a cuddle, she'd hardly even worn the lingerie I'd brought back from the pilgrimage.

I went onto the top balcony, climbed onto the railing and stood there holding onto a down pipe. I watched a patch of oyster-grey water glisten in the sunset and imagined semen jerking, like the first few sputtering drops of water from a sprinkler after a drought.

***

Glenn and I finally got to meet after a phone conversation in which he mentioned he was still experiencing incontinence. I'd been quick to allay his fears and tell him it was still early days.

I drove to Leichhardt and found a park a block back from Norton Street. He was sitting at a table outside Café Sport. My secret confidante looked exactly as I'd envisaged, in his dapper waistcoat and pink-collared shirt. He waved when he recognised me from my brief phone description and we shook hands, ordered coffee and cakes and returned outside on the unspoken assumption traffic noise would ensure privacy.

Glenn told me about his holiday to Hawaii. They'd avoided the famous surf beaches, staying on the 'non-commercial' side of the island, hiring bikes and riding in the hills. Lucy was now planning a trip to America on her own to take part in the Al Gore environmental push. Reading between the lines, I presumed it was also to give Glenn time to recover from the operation.

We talked about everything except secret men's business. When he told me about his IT work, I envisaged geeks sitting around PlayStations inventing updates and apps. I couldn't help liking him despite his political correctness when he criticised smokers a couple of tables away as their delicious smoke wafted down the footpath in our direction.

'Some people still haven't got the message about smoking,' he said. 'It should be banned outside cafés on the footpath as well.'

'I've smoked on and off over my life,' I confessed. 'Luckily I started late because of sport. So I never really got into it until my mid twenties. And I've also had long periods of abstinence over the years and, of course, recently because of the operation. I don't think a bit of passive cigarette smoke in the street can do much harm compared with carbon monoxide from cars.'

There was a flicker of a smile. I'd hesitated before putting my two bob's worth in because, despite feeling I was the larrikin elder here, it was obvious we liked each other. And if anything was going to develop between us there was no point in not being utterly honest. At least we were in accord about not wanting to join the collective prostate cancer clubs, although neither of us had anything against their existence as such.

Glenn mentioned a website he'd found with a link to 'noninvasive' methods for treating the after-effects of prostate cancer surgery. He promised to email his research. I was less than convinced but tried to sound grateful. I'd already seen enough brochures and booklets and stared at enough websites about prostate cancer to last me a lifetime.

'You said you're still experiencing some incontinence?' I said. 'I've pissed my pants too, mate.'

Over the phone he'd sounded almost unconcerned about it. As if it were just another Google Game to master if you knew the right links.

'How long before you stopped being incontinent after your op?' he asked.

'About a month and a half, but it's an individual thing. I wouldn't worry about it.'

'I'm using three pads a day.'

'Did they give you any pre-operation pelvic-floor exercises to do?'

'Not until after the operation.'

'That surprises me. My surgeon's team got me onto it well before the operation.'

My photographic exhibition red dots were still stuck on our stairs as a reminder.

Glenn smiled. 'Maybe I need to get an electronic diary with a beeper. I just forget to do them.'

At the Royal Prince Alfred Hospital on prep day, it had been made very clear to me that the more pelvic-floor exercise you do before the operation the better your chances of not suffering long-term incontinence. I'd heard from my brother in Melbourne that a neighbour of his was *still* incontinent five years after his operation. His only option now was another operation to try and fix a botched job. In the meantime he just had to put up with wearing nappies.

Glenn said he would be taking it up with his surgeon at the next appointment and then we talked about erections or, rather, their lack. I told him Viagra had not had much effect in my case and the possibility that I might have to use a needle for the rest of my life.

'Urologists are not specialists in sexuality,' Glenn said, 'they might know what they know but are not trained about sexuality after the operation. Before the operation my surgeon had me on a low dose of Cialis. It's a phosphodiesterase inhibitor that helps keep erectile tissue from thickening until the nerves heal.'

I smiled at the polysyllabic mumbo-jumbo. But his mention of thickening, the beginning of the end, had me worried. He sipped his tea and continued. 'I've also been seeing a naturopath. He felt my penis a few days ago and told me there was no sign of long-term damage.'

'*My* surgeon never mentioned anything about pills *before* the operation,' I said.

'There's a whole world of knowledge out there that most oncologists don't know about because it's not seen as part of their job to know,' the unflappable pixie said.

In July last year, it had been none other than Glenn's eventual surgeon who'd rung me on my mobile when I was driving to a photography job. The same one who'd wanted Anna and me to meet a couple of his satisfied customers. But we'd found him so run off his feet that he was sweating. I imagined the conveyor belt I'd narrowly avoided. After I pulled over the surgeon had sounded more like a salesman as he offered 'a unique pelvic-floor procedure' as an 'add-on during the operation at no extra cost'. The surgeon who hadn't even advised Glenn to do the basic pelvic-floor exercises before the operation.

So I did wonder about Glenn's moon-faced optimism, and I felt lucky to have chosen the no-frills young traditional surgeon we did. I felt vindicated by his perfect continence record, which I for one had not sullied.

But it was relaxing siting there with Glenn, shooting the breeze. Talking about men's business one-on-one outside the system. Just being with him made me feel almost normal again. I certainly felt lighter as I walked back to my car, aware of having said fuck once too often. Compared with Glenn I *was* almost normal again, medically speaking.

But I wasn't of course. And therein lay the danger. Accepting the consequences of D Day as a natural part of growing old. We had shared the secret in an intimate way. The way sick people forge a bond, and kids cut fingers and mingle blood to belong to the gang.

When I got home I gushed to Anna about Glenn's love of cinema and art but not his strident anti-smoking mind-set. Not that there was anything new about that in this ideologically fashionable age. When I suggested inviting him over for dinner, Anna said she thought it was a bit soon for that. But she was very happy I'd found a male confidante.

16

I was reading an article about Chinese medicine in a magazine in my GP's waiting room. It reminded me of the printout my herbalist Kevin Lu gave me after I'd been unable to conceal my anger at losing my mojo.

> Youth means the temperamental predominance of courage over timidity, of the appetite of adventure over the love of ease. This often exists in a man of sixty more than in a boy of twenty. Nobody grows old by merely living a number of years. We grow old by deserting our ideals...

It had been months since I'd been to see our GP. The last time had been for a referral for a psychologist after Anna's suggestion, when I'd gone home and filled out the forms and promptly did nothing.

This time it was for a referral for a sex specialist. Although my surgeon had offered a specialist within the hospital network whose consultation would have been free – though the medicine is certainly not – I needed as good as it got. That's what my father had always said. Don't muck about. If there's a problem go straight to the top. Anna had offered to help with the cost.

Our GP handed me a card for his recommended sex specialist so promptly it was as if *I'd* been the one advising. As if I was the expert in the field. His alacrity was a good sign. He'd been almost as quick to recommend my surgeon.

I'd asked him a while back to ring my herbalist, given that they spoke the same language. 'Yes, I rang him,' he said, smiling. 'He is doing the Yin and Yang Chinese approach, from the point of view of overall balance. It certainly can't do any harm.'

'Did he tell you what the herbs were exactly?' I asked.

Our GP laughed. 'No, I'm afraid not. On that score we speak different languages. Kevin's treatment is based on ancient ingredients, shall we say. But I'm sure he knows what he's doing.'

Our GP assumed I knew what Yin and Yang meant, as far as any Westerner could. Or I may have used the term in a previous conversation. The important thing was that he thought it worth persevering with my herbalist, Kevin Lu. I produced a tiny pamphlet for the prescription drug that Kevin gave me, when he'd told me it was better than Viagra because it worked well even after a meal and also stayed in the bloodstream for thirty-six hours instead of twelve.

Our GP knew the drug. When he said the strange word, 'Cialis', it dawned on me that it was the same pill Glenn's robotics surgeon prescribed *before* his operation in daily five-milligram dosage. When I mentioned Glenn, the GP said he didn't know about that, but the sex specialist he was referring me to, certainly would.

'In the meantime,' he smiled, 'I'll write you a prescription for the full-strength twenty-milligram Cialis. Worth a shot.'

In the weeks leading to the appointment with the sex specialist I continued to exercise my penis in case I could conjure a miracle. Use it or lose it. In the fetishist white underpants I would bring on the bulge in front of the full-length mirror an hour and a half after taking Cialis. It produced a semblance of an erection that lasted no longer than an orgasm itself. But I fantasised that if I could time it right I might be able to penetrate. I'd tried to let Anna in on my lone pro-active hand, but suspected she was just as happy to wait for Mother Nature to kick back in. Or pragmatic enough to realise that our surgeon hadn't said 'you're probably going to need help' for nothing. I think she kept her own counsel because she was wise enough to realise that talking about sex or its lack, could only make things worse.

Before going to see the sex specialist for the first time, I received an email from Glenn with a long attachment in the kind of objective medical gobbledegook that sexless researchers love to use when talking about *other people:*

> Erectile dysfunction following a prostatectomy remains a significant quality of life issue ... it is estimated to affect 26–100% of patients after

> surgery ... advancements in understanding the anatomy of the prostate and the neurovascular bundles ... the changes of neuropraxis, ischemic and hypoxic insults, fibrotic remodelling apoptosis are all believed to contribute to erectile dysfunction ... the etiologies of nerve neuropraxia include mechanical stretch injury from electrocautery use, and inflammation after surgical trauma ... this neuropraxia can prevent erections and the perpetual lack of erections set up a cascade of deleterious processes ... however the research has yet to be translated into a coherent clinical strategy for penile rehabilitation ... A stringent randomised, double-blinded placebo controlled study was performed ... evaluating the efficacy of daily Sildenafil in men after bilateral nerve sparing radical prostatectomy. This study included 54 men with baseline normal EF and NPTR nocturnal penile tumescence and rigidity with duration of rigidity and of maximal rigidity using plethysmography.

To them we are no more than lab rats with ED. I wondered about Glenn's approach. It was no more than a computer game, an extension of the sixties ethos 'the medium is the message'. To make matters worse he started sending attachments about yogic exercises that purported to help get erections back. A German website wanted you to imagine sitting on a cushion of rice and sucking the grains up into the anus. 'Willing them' by flexing your potency muscles, the pelvic-floor muscles. Accompanied by in-your-face diagrams that stylistically combined German Discipline with Californian Hype. Apparently I should stand with my feet in line with my shoulders and imagine a small cloth draped over my penis, and 'try to move the cloth upwards in the direction of the belly'. In the same contradictory breath I was ordered to 'try harder. It is very important that you listen to your body. Do not force yourself. Simply use strength!'.

There was also pattering, an exercise that involved running on the spot while trying to maintain the maximum speed for thirty seconds and after that 'a series of similar bursts – the circulation of the penis is at its maximum after this strenuous interval training. So therefore please do not take a cold shower after right away but first relax for a certain amount of time'.

Hitler had spoken. I would not obey. Overall I couldn't see much difference between the New Age speak embedded in Glenn's Internet research and the simplistic booklets the hospitals gave out. Stick figures of couples in bed looking like sexless children. The husband with his arm around the wife and idiotic musical notes dancing above the bedhead and the caption: You Can Still Make Music To The Beat of a Different Drum. The accompanying text was in the usual soulless medical matter-of-fact style. Listing the alternative ways of getting an erection, or at least the physical way of getting an artificial erection, which is not quite the same thing. Implants in the scrotum, penile injections, and vacuum pumps. Spelled out in such a singsong style as to lull the unsuspecting bloke into thinking it's no big deal. Just making music to the beat of a different drum, mate. All good. Too easy.

I associated the phrase 'to the beat of a different drum' with the sixties encounter groups. But in fact the derivation of the word 'drum' is from the Tamil word for drummer: 'Of the darkest skin, the lowest caste, *the outcast.*'

Outcast had been a word my mother would use to describe those less fortunate than us. I remember when I was about fifteen. There had been the hint of a psychic skeleton in the family closet when she used that term during a discussion about the family tree, and the painters on her side of the family. But I had to admit to a flicker of desire when I visualised the Germanic lederhosen lap-lap, rising towards my belly button and the will to power in the German Gestalt.

Reality only sank in when I realised that Anna and I had not made proper love in over six months. Seeing the sex specialist might already be too late for me. I started to see how easy it would be to slip into believing it was all part of growing old. Curling up in bed to the beat of books. *There's much more to this beautiful life than sex.*

I was beginning to see why a lot of men would succumb, and go gently into that good night and *not keep trying.* Thanks, Dad.

***

Just the thought of a second post-operative PSA test was enough to trigger the fear all over again. Even though the gland had been removed, the prostate-specific antigen test was the only indicator of cancer cells still in the bloodstream, slowly making their way to the base of the spine. So I always dreaded going to Norton Street for the blood test and the appointment with the surgeon for the results. But I had finally gone there and rolled up my sleeve.

I uncrossed my fingers as I crossed the road outside the clinic and walked to the bookshop. An ethereal male voice registered out of the void, the eccentrically talented busker Anna and I had seen in Balmain when we went out for breakfast after my release from hospital. He was playing the same song. Max Merritt's old classic 'Slipping Away'.

I put two dollars in his guitar case and his gorgeous falsetto followed me all the way to the cinema bookshop until the heavy glass doors closed. I scanned the shelves for Bettina Arndt's new book, *The Sex Diaries.* I'd fortuitously photographed her during a talk at The Sydney Institute. The Institute had employed me as their back-up photographer for a few years, a job that had come indirectly via my photography teaching college. Arndt had opened her talk by stating that men and women needed to make time for sex. She finished by quoting the old hippie mantra *Just do it,* which back then meant burning money, burning your bra, burning your draft card, and making love in the street. Bettina wasn't going that far. Just doing it in your bedroom more often than not was revolutionary enough for her modern mandate. I felt grateful and vindicated when she said: 'I've always thought erections to be the most marvellous things. So I can understand men missing them terribly.'

I found the chapter I was looking for: *Sex After Prostate Cancer Surgery.* The first diary entry jumped off the page. It was 'the sad tale' of a man who'd had the operation four years earlier and was now partially impotent. But he had great support from his wife. His wife had said they needed to make love as much as possible before the operation, 'as things would never be the same'.

That rang a bell. It reminded me of the sex we'd had over the three months between the Melbourne surgeon shocking us into action and the date of the operation.

Another of Bettina's diarists wrote: 'I must have been down, feeling sorry for myself, possibly a bit depressed.'

Possibly?

The old stiff upper lip in place of a stiff penis 'as smooth as a scar', a description of an erection I'd read in a novel. I knew only too well that those poetic words did not apply to flaccid male flesh.

I read on. Another man had found a 'feeling of peace' after he and his wife had been able to make love again 'even though it wasn't the same'.

I thought back to the night my old friend Julian visited, when Anna gave me the number of the prostate cancer 'expert'. After Julian left that night I rang my brother in Melbourne, knowing he'd still be up watching old *Colombo* episodes. I felt like the famous detective himself returning for that last question, just as the suspect is pouring himself a well-deserved scotch. When the detective scratches his head as if it's just occurred to him to ask: 'By the way, how are the erections?'

I could still see Bettina's sensual lips. Her attractive face full of teeth when she smiles. When she says 'erection' and 'penis'. People fidgeting a bit as she mentions 'learning to desire desire'. She was wearing a summery grape-coloured dress with a hint of cleavage. She also chose to say 'masturbation' rather than the bourgeois, post-post Freudian 'self-pleasuring', which makes sex sound about as exciting as cutting your own hair. She admitted to a past error, when she joked about seeing her face on a billboard under the banner *Bettina Arndt Gets It Wrong.* Recent research had proven male sexuality was *not* 'all in the mind'.

It was the last section from her *Sex Diaries* that really hit home. One man had written:

What I find is that having an erection and the need for intercourse isn't a desire or want, it's something driven from deep within ... to be a male and then have this taken from you would be a killer on its own and that is an issue that isn't understood. Thank you for spotlighting the fact that men actually have issues and there are emotions attached to them.

It may not have been forensic Freud, but I knew exactly what that man in the street was getting at.

17

We drove in nervous silence to see the sex specialist and parked in a street near a redbrick building reminiscent of the VD clinics in Melbourne, circa the seventies in my case. I wondered whether we'd be left alone after learning how to inject. Whether I would be able to do it in the special room to the scent of aromatic oils.

Anna took the lift. I took to the stairs. We met up on the next floor and walked along a blue-carpeted corridor past doors advertising various specialists, including a sexual health psychologist.

The waiting room seemed claustrophobically small, as small as my dick felt under the cloud of nervous anticipation of having to flop it out for the dick doctor. A solitary gent sat in the corner fiddling on some device. I went through to reception and got a cup of cold water from a dispenser to kill time while waiting for the secretary to finish her interminable conversation with a potential client. After filling in the paperwork I re-joined Anna in the waiting room. The other man was poring at his device with both thumbs, while the radio pumped out 'round the clock' news. Anna had found a newspaper and was doing the Sudoku. In the dim windowless room, the air felt heavy with the collective memory of flaccid dicks

By the time the sex specialist's head appeared between the curtains and called my name, I had determined to forget my fear and get my old nerve back. He reminded me of a cuddly bear in a collared shirt, no tie, and laundered faded-blue jeans. We followed him to a room where he indicated a couple of chairs on the other side of a large desk, neat piles of paper on the table next to his computer, and shelves filled with books and fat ring-binders.

I'd been expecting someone in a white coat with a clinical aura to boot. But he presented with a down-to-earth bedside manner. A mannequin, similar to the Picasso doll in the Melbourne surgeon's consultation room, was used to punctuate his spiel about the prostate. He asked how my erections had been before surgery. The same question they all asked. And he made sure he addressed Anna, who didn't let me down. She said I'd been virile. I said my erections came naturally enough, but didn't mention sometimes *too* naturally. I could sometimes start to get hard for no particular reason in my car, waiting for traffic lights to change.

The sex specialist referred to the paperwork sent by my surgeon and reiterated what I'd first heard from our GP nine months ago: 'Your surgeon is known for his nerve-sparing abilities.'

So far, so good.

'But you're now seven months on from your radical prostatectomy and you need to know that your clock is ticking,' he said, continuing to hold my gaze with his pragmatic, no-bullshit attitude.

'I want you to take low-grade five milligram Cialis for the next twelve months on a daily basis. They are to help bring back your nocturnal erections, which in turn will help stave off any lasting thickening in the erectile tissue. I would've had you on a course of low dosage Cialis before the operation if it had been up to me. Do you any have health insurance?'

'No.'

'No matter, you don't really save much even if you are on private. I'll give you some information about an on-line place where you can get it cheaper. It's a reputable source unlike the many charlatans out there on the World Wide Web. Any questions thus far?'

'I've been taking Viagra and Cialis, the strongest dose in each case and they're pretty expensive, four tablets for about eighty dollars. I could easily go broke.'

I could almost feel Anna holding her tongue, knowing that I prided myself on not bludging off her for my medical expenses even if I was taxing her emotional reserves.

'A packet of these five milligram Cialis taken on a daily basis will cost about two hundred bucks but will last you a month. Has Viagra had any effect on your erections?'

'They've caused a swelling but only if I do some serious masturbation,' I said. Feeling despair on the rise, the doubts kicking in again.

He didn't bat an eyelid.

'As I've said, Cialis will help restore your nocturnal erections by increasing the blood flow on a daily basis. This will hasten your recovery, because the longer the erectile tissue remains dormant, the less likely it is that your erections will ever return. Statistically you've got about another eighteen months before your clock stops ticking.' I wondered how many times he'd slipped up and said cock instead of clock. 'Your surgeon has recommended that you learn how to inject into your penis,' he said, turning to Anna who was taking notes.

Then sensing that I was not entirely over the moon, he looked back at me. 'The drug is a three-stroke mix called Caverject. One of the components is for the pain factor. You can't get it through the Royal Prince Alfred, so it's a bit more expensive. But you'll be pleased to hear that injecting not only aids the rehabilitation process, you'll be able to have sex again.'

I'd perked up a bit at the mention of sex.

'From what you've told me regarding your erectile capability, such as it is at this stage, it's clear your surgeon saved some of your nerve bundles – otherwise there would be no swelling at all, with or without Viagra.'

He said I should make another appointment for him to teach me how to self-inject. I had a fleeting thought about whether he was thinking of capital S or small s when he used the term self-inject. Whether he really understood that it was the potential resurrection of the male Self rather than just creating the mechanical function.

But I'd had a reprieve. I wouldn't be putting cold steel into the old boy today.

'I'll have to work out the correct mixture in your case and I'll also warn you about some of the potential side effects of injecting. One is that an erection might hang around too long. The medical term for it is a priapism.' He laughed: 'Given where you're at right now, that no doubt sounds like heaven. But I can assure you you'll get pretty sick of it after six hours.'

I sat there in nervous silence not daring to look at Anna. Then I remembered that I'd brought printouts of Glenn's Internet research to ask about the vacuum pump and the German yoga exercises.

He grinned when I flourished the printouts with accompanying diagrams.

'Total bullshit. As far as the pump goes – it circulates the wrong blood in your case. From the veins instead of freshly oxygenated arterial blood.'

Glenn had recently visited The Tool Shed in Darlinghurst where he'd bought a pump from some very helpful homosexual shop assistants. But when he'd gone home to put it on it was, he said with a smile, big enough for an elephant. You had to love Glenn's sense of humour beneath his naïve faith in the informational highway. But he had been spot on. This sex specialist, an associate professor of medicine no less, knew what he was talking about. Not to forget our GP who seemed to have the happy knack of recommending the best specialists despite the shocking words that had been yelled over the phone by the president of the Secret Men's Club the night Julian turned up unexpectedly from overseas: 'He should be taken outside and shot' – a sentiment that had probably contributed to my mistrust of those organisations ever since.

The sex doctor insisted Anna should come next time too. When he would teach me how to inject with the 'jungle juice'. I looked around the Bear's consultation room for any sign of the curtained-off candle-lit room where, after injecting, we'd presumably be left to our own devices.

***

A few days later, there was an untimely newspaper headline: 'Experts Question Value of Prostate Cancer Test.' A book had been published with the clichéd, but very effective title: *Let Sleeping Dogs Lie,* co-authored by a professor of public health from the University of Sydney no less.

I read it with horror: 'The PSA test cannot distinguish deadly cancers from those that will not cause a problem. Men treated for those cancers – through surgery or radiation – can often become impotent or incontinent.'

The article went on: 'Half of NSW's biggest names in cancer and health research were old enough to have regular testing, but chose not to do so. Of eight who agreed to comment, five said they would not undergo regular PSA testing. Five other experts refused to comment.'

An associate professor from Westmead Millennium Institute of Medical Research had said that 'at best PSA testing would only give you a very small chance of not dying early'. Other experts were quoted including oncologists, surgeons, statisticians and Cancer Council notables.

The catchy title *Let Sleeping Dogs Lie* would help sell the horrid book because that's exactly what a man wanted to hear. Exactly what most men would rather do than risk knowing. Excellent marketing. The old debate was a bit old for me.

But then in Monday's Letters to the Editor, a contributor had written that Bettina Arndt had 'got it all wrong' about the difference between the funding women receive for reconstruction after breast cancer treatment and what is available for men after prostate cancer treatment: 'Prostate cancer is a relatively benign cancer, often not needing surgery or chemotherapy.' She had completely missed Bettina's point. What Bettina had actually said was, 'women receive far more funding for breast reconstruction than the government makes available for the essential treatments *necessary for men's well being*'. And thankfully a few letters took issue with the woman who'd accused Bettina of getting it all wrong including one brave man who replied: 'Over eight years I have had surgery, radiotherapy, and hormone treatments that produced physical and emotional effects no less profound than the loss of a breast, and caused me to retire as a senior doctor in a teaching hospital.'

Nevertheless, this rotten article implied that I should've listened to my inner voice instead of being panicked into it by the Melbourne oncologist.

Then I had a flash of logical insight: *The sensationalist article had omitted to mention anything about the definitive bloody biopsy test!*

My panic cleared. It dawned on me that the glaring omission had been quite deliberate. It was all about selling newspapers. Only *one* letter had come from an expert who'd actually *had* prostate cancer surgery himself. 'I made sure I chose a surgeon who'd specialised in prostate surgery to minimise the chance of side effects.'

He also spelt out recent advances in prostate cancer statistics and new diagnostic tools. He'd witnessed the distressing deaths of men in their forties and fifties from prostate cancer, and was grateful he'd made an informed decision to have the PSA test to minimise the risk of 'a similar fate'. When I saw the name at the bottom of the letter I was shocked. It was the same radiology specialist I'd contacted two years earlier at the behest of a member of Anna's family, who just happened to be a professor with a doctorate in 'post cancer quality of life'.

In the first month after my diagnosis, Anna and I visited her at her home where she provided detailed, up-to-the moment research, including graphs about outcomes for various treatments for prostate cancer correlated to variables such as age, PSA, and biopsy Gleason scores.

I decided to give the radiologist another ring. I came straight to the point and after re-introducing myself and mentioning having read the article, I asked about his sex life. And he came straight to the point too. He said it was non-existent. He and his wife had made the decision not to go down any of the radical rehab paths such as injecting, or the vacuum pump, or the implant. They all seemed 'too much bother'. He sounded calm, very matter of fact.

I thanked him for his time. The instant I hung up, I decided he sounded like a good man who gives up too easily.

***

I'd been putting off going to the therapist. I read the GP's Patient Plan copy again, the one I'd filled out and then nearly thrown out.

Under *Patient Needs/Main Issues:* 'He is upset about the loss of erections and the possible necessity for the Caverject penile injections for the rest of his life.'

Under *Goals:* 'He wants to feel at peace about the decision over the prostate treatment.'

Under *Treatments* the GP had scrawled: 'Continue to be active by playing tennis, develop strategies with local psychologist.'

I went there straight after Saturday morning tennis. The clinic was within walking distance of home so I could have gone after tennis, a shower and a spruce up. But going directly, still in my tennis gear, seemed to downplay it all.

I mounted a wooden staircase to his tiny room overlooking a courtyard, with a window framing a pepper tree. He was young, about forty, compared with the bearded sage-like Freudian figure of my imagination, and wore a humble green cardigan that looked like a family heirloom.

I sat down on a plain chair opposite his identical chair, no table between 'expert' and patient. He referred to my GP's report and asked how I'd been going since filling out the forms he'd received months ago. It seemed unlikely that this young guy could possibly understand. I said I was suspicious of the questionnaire's categories in the first place. They didn't apply to my situation, knowing he would've read the final report from the GP: 'Suffering from adjustment disorder with depression.'

'I will probably have to use a needle to inject a drug called Caverject into my penis to have sex,' I said. Cutting to the un-Freudian fucking chase.

'Because of the prostate surgery, yes of course,' he carried on, unfazed.

'That's right, although I can still masturbate and get a phantom erection and have an orgasm.'

I told him I agreed with my GP that I was having difficulty accepting the loss of natural erections. I was prepared to give the needle a go. But I was still hoping natural erections would eventually return. I said I occasionally felt as if I'd made the wrong decision after being panicked into it by the Melbourne surgeon.

He told me his father had the operation and the Caverject had been stored in the fridge in a white box for years. This information was a bombshell to me. By proxy he himself had direct personal experience just by mentioning 'the white box' in his father's fridge. I told him I was writing a book about it. I told him that if nothing else, politicians needed to know the cost of rehabilitation for men after prostate surgery, we were not all on obscene corporate wages, some of us still had to shop at BI-LO. I told him it also needed to be said that men's cancer isn't just about physical rehabilitation but mental health.

The young therapist took my rant in his stride. There was something about him, an understanding beyond his years. 'Have you got a title for your book yet?' he said.

'*The Needle and the Damage Done,* the Neil Young song.'

He hardly missed a beat, 'How about *The Needle* for *the Damage Done?*'

'I like it,' I said.

'A philosopher's system of thought always arises from autobiography,' he said. 'Sartre's idea of freedom is defined as "taking responsibility". A term misused in pop psychology these days. Sartre meant becoming the author of the design of your life.'

A bird alighted on a branch outside the window and for a moment I imagined it was my father, flying in the face of facts.

I shook the therapist's hand. At the door I turned to him and said, 'I want you to know that even if I don't come back, it certainly won't be because of *you.* I trust you entirely.'

As I walked out of the clinic I thought about his last words: 'I can help you with the sexual fantasy issues you mentioned. I specialise in sexual communication between couples.'

I walked home pleased to see people in cafés reading the Saturday papers and drinking coffee. Several times I stopped to look up at the sulphur-crested cockatoos shrieking from the crucifix-tops of telegraph poles and then dive-bombing the traffic snarl along Victoria Road.

When I got home I imagined the fridge door automatically flying open.

***

We were back in the sex specialist's waiting room listening to the round-the-clock news. I was resigned to the needle as a way of using it or losing it, as a bridge to help Mother Nature kick back in after a year or so. Follow the treatment to its logical conclusion.

I thought of how I'd wrecked everything the day we'd gone to the pub to celebrate the results of the wonderful first postoperative PSA test. When it ended in tears because I'd said, 'I wish I'd never met him.' And when I disappeared into a fug of depression the day at the beach, for no good reason. The arguments about wanting Anna to spend less time at her mum's in order to spend more time on my sexual rehabilitation.

I had no idea why Anna was honouring the dick doctor's wish that she be there. I suspected it was pity. Either that or she wanted to put an end to the suffocating effect the last six months had had on *her* life.

It also occurred to me that it wasn't in her nature not to throw herself in where angels fear to tread. All I wanted to do now was *love her.* The associate professor's statuesque head appeared at the gap in the curtain. He called my name. Staring at the computer screen, he stated where we'd left off last time. He asked if the low-dose Cialis had produced any improvement in my erections.

'I've woken a couple of times with a sort of erection.'

He smiled: 'What do you mean by "sort of"?'

'It feels like bordering on stiffening. For about three seconds. It always seems to coincide with waking up to urinate during the night. Or when I wear jocks to bed.'

He looked me in the eye. 'It would have nothing to do with the desire to urinate. That would be pure coincidence,' he said. 'And as far as the underpants go that could be static electricity?' From the lop-sided smile and the deliberate upwards inflection it was obvious he was humouring me. But I still believed it all had something to do with it. Perhaps 'the science' was not so set in cement as the experts and specialists thought. There may still be an unknown in the equation. But we all laughed. 'It's good to see you smile,' he said. 'Last time you looked shit-scared.'

His in-your-face language was the other thing I liked about this bear of a man, quite apart from his honesty. 'I *was* shit-scared,' I said, feeling the weight lift in that simple admission. I looked him in the eye instead of jerking my gaze all over the place as I had last time.

The time had come.

He invited us to come closer to his desk and pointed to a cross-section of the penis. He pointed out the corpus cavernosum, the erectile tissue in the side of the penis where you could inject without harming the urethra. Like a magician pulling a rabbit out of a hat, he flourished a tiny bottle of colourless 'jungle juice'. He demonstrated the sterilisation of the phial's dark grey porous top with an alcohol swab and then how to get the stuff into the syringe to the right dosage; in my case twelve milligrams – half the maximum dosage. I felt almost lucky.

The syringe was much smaller than I'd imagined. He used his arm to show how to swab the penis after the injection and then, without further ado, led me to a chair and told me to take off my jeans and undies. He sat beside me on another chair, told me to inject my penis.

It all happened so quickly that before I knew it he was pointing out a freckle on the side of my dick I'd never noticed before. He said it would become my 'landmark'.

After I'd successfully injected and withdrawn and swabbed he grinned and owned up.

It was only water.

But I'd passed with flying colours and he commended me on my technique.

I told him he probably said that to all his men friends. He laughed and I took Anna's hand, feeling a bit ridiculous and a bit proud.

'I think it's worth your while paying the extra, over and above what you'd get through the Royal Prince Alfred. It will cost $175, including enough needles to last you about six months. So that's three dollars a shot, thirty cents an inch.'

He gave another droll grin while my brain raced to do the maths. Based on the figures, he was talking a ten-inch erection.

'The rule of thumb for Caverject is six months in the fridge, six weeks out,' he said, still waiting for me to get back about the maths.

'If your erection takes longer than two hours to go down, take a couple of Sudafed tablets and go for a long walk. Only if it takes longer than ten hours, should you ring me on my private number.'

He spoke into a high-tech device that converted speech into a memo stored in his computer. 'Even if the injections don't ultimately bring back your erections after about eighteen months,' he said, 'that's not the end of the world either. A patient of mine in his seventies has been successfully injecting himself for over twenty years.'

He told me to make an appointment to see him again in a month. We were halfway out the door when he added, 'And if you get an erection from the water, ring me and I'll bottle it.'

On the way back to the car I stopped Anna in her tracks and kissed her. Really kissed her. Out in the open for all to see. It was a kiss that had nothing to do with sex or bed.

18

I was about to go in the front door after returning from the pool when I noticed a package behind one of the rubbish bins on the front veranda. It was swathed in an Egyptian mummy's worth of heavy duct tape and I instantly knew. It was unlabelled, very discreet.

The jungle juice had arrived.

I tore the tape off in the kitchen and unwound the packaging. The same polystyrene box the psychologist had mentioned his father kept in his fridge. It was not much bigger than a lunchbox. Inside was a plastic bag of ice cubes that had mostly melted, the phial of jungle juice, and packets of needles. I felt a huge sense of relief and gratitude for the fast delivery, the ice cubes further proof that they really cared. That it wasn't just a money-making operation. The lack of fanfare and the less than ideal spot behind the rubbish bin didn't detract from their professionalism at all.

There were syringes in six sealed plastic bags and dozens of alcohol swabs. I made space in the fridge, wondering if Anna would complain about the white box taking up food space. To think that a year ago I'd turned white myself just hearing the oncologists mention that if worse came to worst, I would still be able to get an erection by sticking a needle into my dick. I remembered how they viewed the final solution as no more than a Dada theatre version of treating diabetes.

As I deposited the polystyrene box amongst pasta sauces and jars of pickles, my future sexual life seemed frozen in time. It had all sounded okay in theory at the dick doctor's clinic. Injecting the water was innocuous enough, but having the real drug safely stashed away in the fridge – power failures notwithstanding – made it all suddenly set in cement, my soul on ice.

I counted the needles in a bag. Twelve. Six months for the jungle juice to remain potent. I did the sums. About three fucks a week. I sat there at the kitchen table and tried to avoid looking at the graphic diagram of how to inject, the old boy pulled over a schematic thigh like a useless sausage, sad-sack testicles dangling.

The heading said: 'Penile Injection With Penis Stretched Over Thigh.'

I wondered whether my balls would be affected by the injections – would they tighten as natural nuts did nearing orgasm, or remain deflated party balloons? I knew I would still have dry orgasms – that part of the modern miracle was nonnegotiable. I opened the fridge again. The new arrival was still there. I hadn't dreamt it. The white elephant was made of the same material as my first Malibu surfboard, which had also symbolised freedom. I thought about putting a label on it, regressing to communal household politics where everyone had his or her separate food items labelled upon pain of death should anyone feel *too* communally inclined.

But overall I felt a wave of relief knowing the thimble-sized phial containing the tri-mix magic was now in my fridge, even staring you in the face upon opening the door. I imagined needing easy access to avoid searching through jars of pickles and glad-wrapped leftovers that would be counter productive for having sex as smoothly as possible under my circumstances.

The specialist had mentioned placing a needle and swab near the bed to make it more natural, akin to a photographer pre-focusing when the automatic system freezes up. But I was more worried about the magic stuff losing its potency out of the fridge. Perhaps after taking the five-milligram Cialis for a couple of months, it might be easier, might all happen without performance anxiety.

I got the dick doc's pamphlet out and took the phial from the fridge and opened a bag of needles. There was a diagram of an upside-down cross that reminded me of the crucifixion. I sat at the kitchen table and re-read the instructions for loading a syringe: 'The head of the penis is firmly grasped between the thumb and the forefingers and the penis is firmly stretched obliquely over the thigh...'

The ninth step in the pamphlet's ten-step program instructed me to apply an alcohol swab to the site for about a minute after withdrawing the needle, longer if there was bleeding. I tried to imagine waking in the morning feeling horny, in the mind at least, and how all this rigmarole would destroy the spontaneity. But at least I'd hopefully be able to make love to Anna again.

I was about to finally load my first needle in anticipation of having sex with Anna the minute she walked in the door, when the prescient cat leapt onto my lap making the most of it before my groin had time to stir.

I put her on the floor and went to the bathroom to wash my hands. When I came back she stayed at my feet, supervising operations, pleased that I was finally getting on with life. Buoyed by her clairvoyant abilities and crackling purr, I removed the plastic stopper from the syringe's plunger. With the tricky push-pull action I removed the Hare Krishna-orange cap from the gunmetal grey needle, and without mercy stabbed the phial's porous top, then struggled to invert it all and draw the stuff into the syringe without snapping the damn thing in two with my clumsy manhandling. It had seemed a breeze in the dick doctor's clinic but here midst domestic familiarity I felt like a klutz.

After three attempts I hoped I'd succeeded in excluding the last of the air bubbles – only to find out later that I'd imagined them, just tiny imperfections resembling air bubbles.

I loaded three more needles and put everything back in the fridge, then prepared enough pasta for two. I kept the sauce simple: two tins of tomatoes, half an eggplant salted and washed, a clove of chopped garlic and *de rigueur* dried basil. Sitting on the deck I watched the avocado tree trembling and glistening in a sudden tropical downpour.

I waited for Anna in a state of nervous anticipation. I had turned the lamp towards the curtains to soften the light and put on the television without the sound and closed the double balcony doors to keep everything womb-like. When I heard her arrive, I raced downstairs. We kissed in the kitchen. I told her about the delivery. 'It came by courier. There's *jungle juice* in the fridge now,' I said, pouring two glasses of wine.

'That was quick,' Anna said.

She plonked her bag down and took the glass of wine. She smiled at me and we toasted.

'Here's to not going gently into that good night,' I said

'Here's to *us,*' she said and we clinked glasses.

I opened the fridge and took out the white box and showed her its alchemical contents. 'Let's eat later. See you up there?'

She kissed me. 'See you up there in a few minutes.'

I could feel her lips still on mine as I went back to the bedroom, a feeling worth more than money could buy. But knowing I was about to do what had been impossible for close to a year made me nervous. I stood in front of the computer and flicked at the shape in my underpants, mentally preparing for the jab. Just as I had torn open the swab, Anna came in wearing her charcoal-grey and dust-rose satin knickers. She lay down on the bed behind me in the candlelight. I had to concentrate on what I was doing but even the scent of the ether was erotic to my wide-open imagination. I uncapped the syringe and dropped my undies, found the dick doctor's freckle, and gently pushed the needle in. Then went totally blank before remembering to depress the plunger. I withdrew the needle and put the ethereal tool on the table, feeling slightly wobbly on my legs at the palpable apprehension of sex again. I stood there with the swab on the injection site as the swelling came on and then the old familiar hardening. Without guilt I pulled my white jocks back on to accentuate the tent pole being raised up again. She was making tiny circular motions with her fingers as I walked over, protruding. For her I stood by the bed and felt myself up. Then I lay beside her and we kissed until the old urgency was irresistible and I entered her for the first time in nine months in chiaroscuro candlelight, seeing her beautiful eyelashes turn into blue shadows, feeling confident strokes like velvet, trying to slow everything down.

Anna told me to just go for it.

I was amazed afterwards. Amazed we'd finally broken the spell cast over us too long. I asked her if she'd come. 'Couldn't you tell? You felt as good as ever.'

'Really? So did you,' I said. I was barely able to put two words together. Out of my mind like a schoolboy who has had his first sexual triumph.

We stayed united. I didn't miss ejaculating at all. The orgasm itself was enough. As good as before, for both of us, thank God.

I felt alive for the first time since the diagnosis, cushioning her head on my chest and feeling the stress and anxiety of the last twelve months draining away as she drifted off to sleep. She looked serene, unsullied by my bad karma at last.

I went downstairs to the toilet and after pushing my erection inside the bowl sat there with an overriding sense of relief. After softening a bit, I urinated easily.

I had made love to her again! Nothing else medical mattered.

Upstairs I blew out the candle and lay there in conjugal darkness, conjuring up the surf beach south of Adelaide where my father used to take me.

Dripping up the beach then walking the path to Dad's car, looking back on paradise to the perfect lines of swell with a last surfer flying across the face of a wave. After that, feeling happy enough to die.

I was still erect, but sex can handle contradictions. It's a spider's thread in the moonlight, easily broken, then back in the morning with the dew. I bent both knees up under the sheets to take the pressure off and lay there. A bus pulled in. I listened to it rumble off into the night.

***

Over Easter Anna went to the Southern Highlands to stay with old friends she hadn't seen since my diagnosis. She'd left one of her endearing notes on the kitchen table: 'Bye my heavenly, sexy man. Hope you have a lovely relaxing few days. See you sometime Monday.'

At the bottom she asked if I could cook some of the salmon she'd bought at the market and take it over to her mum's that night. Because of my mother-in-law's macular condition she could no longer read her beloved books and had to use the Blind Society's talking books service. She spent a lot of her life in bed because of her debilitating knees and back, and the eye condition. She usually had several nights' worth of lettuce and egg sandwiches stowed in the fridge, care of Anna. She always appreciated my fish – kept warm on a plate wrapped in Glad Wrap – when it arrived on her doorstep.

She was a great talker and took an interest in other people's lives. Despite probably wanting a richer de facto son-in-law, we got along just fine. She could still wring a conversation out of the smell of an oily rag. I could make her laugh and she could do the same for me. Neither of us suffered fools gladly and we both supported the underdog.

I parked in the cul-de-sac and walked towards the orange glow, behind which she would be ensconced in bed listening to an audio book. Or sitting on the edge of her recliner a foot from the television screen. The sliding door at the side of the house led straight into her bedroom, relocated downstairs because of her buggered eighty-year-old legs and, as usual, unlocked. There she was, miles away, plugged in. I slid the door open, she became aware of my presence and took the earplugs out.

'Meals on Wheels at your disposal,' I said.

'Oh you are funny,' she said, turning the cassette player off and struggling to surface in a sea of pillows like the survivor of a shipwreck. I sat on the edge of her bed and we held hands. For a moment I was tempted to tell her everything. She knew about the prostate cancer and was happy to keep it in the past tense. Anna had not intruded into male taboo territory with her mum. I had the feeling the wise old owl knew that we were okay, sort of.

I took the fish to the kitchen and dished up, while she threw on a gown and took off to the lounge room to watch the news. A part of me wanted to spill the beans because my mum was dead. But I'd always held back. What good would it do? She would only pity me and understandably want something better for her youngest daughter. I couldn't blame my substitute mum preferring stoicism. She was a Churchill woman after all. I had fought the good fight.

After taking the meal over to her on the TV tray, she more or less shooed me out. I still had to go home and cook the rest of the salmon for myself. I slid the door closed and walked to my car feeling guilty I hadn't stayed longer. She couldn't see enough to know if I was lying, or not. Ever since the PSA test I had said I was fine whenever she asked, bringing her face up closer to see me more clearly.

I drove down the tree-lined street imagining books and classical music from the chinks of warm light between drawn curtains. I drove back imagining my mum, after I'd told her everything. She would say, 'Look after her, Pete.'

I left Anna's note on the kitchen table and read it every day over Easter while I worked on a photography job for a client who'd hired me to take product shots for his business. He refurbished ATMs that were then installed in convenience stores all over Sydney. I'd confided in him because we were the same age and shared similar counter-cultural backgrounds from the sixties and seventies. He'd told me about a mate of his whose PSA readings had been 'through the roof' for years. Who refused to have the biopsy test because after a lot of research, had come to the conclusion prostate cancer was nature's way of consigning the organ to obsolescence, once its reproductive function was over. I'd met my client's mate a few times and he'd struck me as being mentally very sharp indeed. Nearly seventy, he had decided sex for its own sake was less important than being able to run his travel agency business and go on regular overseas holidays.

He died about six months after I'd first heard about him. It spread to his spine. I almost didn't tell Anna. I was ashamed to feel vindicated about the most difficult decision I'd ever made in my life. But she immediately said, 'You see, we *did* do the right thing.'

Glenn rang on Easter Monday to make a date for coffee when he got back from his parents' shack on the south coast. He said he was back at work but wasn't happy about it. A letter from his oncologist had been misdirected to his workplace while he was on sick leave. One of his colleagues opened it. Now everyone in the office knew. I remember Anna telling me about a friend of hers who knew a man who'd had the operation and found himself on a tightrope – on the one hand wanting his friends to ask him how he was, but on the other not wanting to talk about it at all. I knew that one all too well. I commiserated with Glenn and told him not to let it get to him. I said I'd ring him about coffee when we got back from Bundeena. Where Anna had booked a place on the beach to celebrate my sixtieth birthday.

Author's note

The decision to have the prostatectomy in the hope of a longer life – but with almost unavoidable collateral damage – is the hardest decision I have made. It is a man's dilemma, his worst nightmare, and this book is my attempt to come to terms with it.

I am seven years on from the operation – and those first tentative jottings on beaches and buses and hotel beds in the moleskin diary Anna gave me for Christmas. I wrote 'I am turning into my book' in an early draft. But I kept writing. My mother told me that as a young boy I rose early and danced barefoot on the lawn, and gradually that life force returned.

Sometimes I wish I had held my tongue and stayed true to the stoic silence society expects, even *honours* in its menfolk, propagating the myth that men don't express their feelings. But I, after building and then setting off on my raft of emotions, sailed on.

My father believed in, and handed down, the maxim 'Blood is thicker than water'. I am in touch with interstate and overseas family members, visiting them whenever I can. Once again I am seaworthy, no longer the shipwreck that washed up on the shores of my siblings' homes.

During the writing of this book I read *The Courage To Be* by the existential theologian Paul Tillich. It kept me going when I was about to give up the writing battle. After I made the mistake of letting slip I was writing a book about the trauma I'd experienced, I was advised against it. Dwelling on it would only bring it all up again, I was told. But I didn't care. Other well-meaning people advised 'What doesn't kill you, makes you stronger'. But the first thoughts written in the moleskin did more good than any such philosophic insight. My writing was akin to a trapeze artist's balancing pole, it saved me from falling into the void.

I would like to thank those without whom this book would not have risen from the dead: Richard Walsh, who was inspired by my book and found the end by knocking out the last chapters; Varuna, where I was given the confidence to persevere; Jo, who helped with the initial editing and inspired me to keep going; and my editor, Julia Beaven, for her ear and eye for detail and alternative nuances, her unerring thoroughness, and her inspirational spirit.

Postscript

Peter finished writing this book in a tiny fisherman's cottage in Cornwall where we had started a two-year sabbatical, intending to travel and pursue creative projects. During the first months he worked closely with his editor Julia Beaven from Wakefield Press on the final edit of this memoir. Peter's health was robust. His PSA results continued to be negligible, we had a healthy sex life and his old boyishly enthusiastic self had returned. In typical style, he'd thrown himself into writing a new book and swimming two laps of the bay, even through winter.

In June 2015, barely a week after completing the edit of this book, Peter had a seizure while playing tennis. Scans revealed a growth in the centre of his brain. Yet again we found ourselves in a surgeon's waiting room with our hearts in our mouths. It was the worst possible news: Grade IV glioblastoma, aggressive, inoperable, terminal, with a prognosis from one to three years. The surgeon stressed this was a primary cancer, not a secondary from the prostate cancer, something completely unconnected. Peter had simply been unlucky – one cell had gone haywire for reasons unknown.

How to live after such a sentence? Horror-struck, we staggered back to our cottage, clung to each other and howled for days. After that we started to make plans. As with his prostate cancer, Peter decided to undergo the recommended treatment and try a range of adjunct alternative therapies. We opted to stay in England for another year and resolved to live as fully as we could, mining each day for enjoyment.

Peter sailed through six weeks of chemotherapy and radiotherapy but barely a month later he suffered multiple seizures that were severe and sustained. He awoke from a coma drastically weakened with a catastrophic brain injury. Too late to return to Sydney, Peter came back to the cottage with me to die.

These last six months were intensely lived by us both. Peter was able to say goodbye to his beloved daughter and a host of friends and family who flew across to be with him. We received magnificent support from a local GP, palliative care nurse and a range of carers who gave me respite. We felt the gamut of terror, rage, grief and sadness, yet throughout were sustained by a deep enjoyment of one another's company that had connected us like a golden thread since we'd first met. To our surprise we discovered that we could still laugh and find richness in these days. And as with most things in life, Peter faced death head on. I was with Peter when he died in the early hours of a June morning, with the gulls making their first calls of the day.

Jo Wing, September 2016

Back Cover Material

'If you do nothing it will *kill* you!' thundered the surgeon. Peter Endersbee, musician, photographer, surfer and former football star, was diagnosed with prostate cancer and confronted that terrifying male dilemma – proceed with a radical prostatectomy and face the prospect of impotence, or wait and see.

We all have a story; many men have a prostate cancer story. But stoic silence in the face of a threat to male identity has been a time-honoured option. In *Taking a Punt,* Peter Endersbee breaks the silence to share the story of the aftermath of a surgery that threatened his identity, providing a voice for men facing the dilemma – and for the baffled women in their lives. For at its heart, *Taking a Punt* is a love story, and a celebration of the courage to remain a sexual being.

Frequently very confronting, as a story of prostate cancer must be, but also moving, disturbing and convincing. BRIAN MATTHEWS

A book for all the men who have real trouble sharing their thoughts and feelings and then get overwhelmed in the face of that initial raised PSA. Not to mention their wives/partners who suffer with them. JUDY KENT

For one who has experienced the aftermath of this men's cancer, Taking A Punt is a must read. Peter

Endersbee has provided an incredible insight into the physical, emotional and social impacts this insidious disease has on so many men. DAVID PARKIN, OAM

This is a compelling, confrontingly honest, totally absorbing book. Every man (and his partner) must read it. GRAHAM CORNESEWS

'Long before Eddie Betts, it was Peter Endersbee's pocket', writes Bruce McAvaney.

'That grand final, those two checkside goals, moments of football magic still vivid after all these years.'

Peter Endersbee completed an Arts degree (Hons) in literature and drama at Flinders University, and at the same time was a Sturt footballer during its 'Golden Era' of five consecutive premierships, playing in the last three and kicking two legendary checkside goals in 1968.

Made in the USA
Coppell, TX
05 November 2026

11299185R00127